Waiting at the Gate:
Creativity and Hope
in the Nursing Home

Waiting at the Gate: Creativity and Hope in the Nursing Home

Susan L. Sandel
David Read Johnson

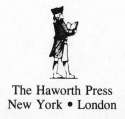

The Haworth Press
New York • London

Waiting at The Gate: Creativity and Hope in the Nursing Home has also been published as *Activities, Adaptation & Aging*, Volume 9, Number 3, Spring 1987.

The Haworth Press, Inc., 12 West 32 Street, New York, NY 10001
EUROSPAN/Haworth, 3 Henrietta Street, London WC2E 8LU England

Library of Congress Cataloging-in-Publication Data

Sandel, Susan L.
   Waiting at the gate.

   Bibliography: p.
   Includes index.
   1. Nursing homes—Recreational activities. 2. Movement therapy. 3. Drama—Therapeutic use. I. Johnson, David Read. II. Title. [DNLM: 1. Dance Therapy—in old age. 2. Homes for the Aged. 3. Literature. 4. Nursing Homes. WT 27.1 S214w]
RA999.R42S26   1987   615.8'51'0880565   87-7428
ISBN 0-86656-631-7
ISBN 0-86656-710-0 (pbk.)

**We dedicate this book
to our grandparents.**

*Sing me a farewell song,
A canticle of life,
For I am leaving land,
And taking space to wife.*

*Into the rising wind
I'll shout the ecstasy.
Echoes will answer back,
I am where I wished to be.*

Wynne Rettger Lewis

About the Authors

SUSAN L. SANDEL, PHD, ADTR, is the Administrator of the New Haven Convalescent Center and a Certified Fellow of the American College of Health Care Administrators. She is a Charter Member of the American Dance Therapy Association and a member of the Academy of Registered Dance Therapists. She is a faculty member at the University of New Haven where she teaches psychology/gerontology courses.

Dr. Sandel developed her movement therapy approach with the elderly at the Sound View Specialized Care Center, West Haven, CT. Her work there is featured in a film produced by the American Dance Therapy Association titled, *Dance Therapy: The Power of Movement.* She has appeared on the NBC *Today* show and *Prime of Your Life*.

Dr. Sandel is on the editorial boards of the *Journal of Long-Term Care Administration* and the *American Journal of Dance Therapy*. She writes a monthly column on issues in long-term care for *Senior News*, a senior citizen newspaper.

Dr. Sandel earned her BA degree from Barnard College, her MA from Goddard College, and her PhD from Union Graduate School.

DAVID READ JOHNSON, PhD, RDT, is a Clinical Psychologist at the West Haven Veterans' Administration Medical Center. He is an Assistant Clinical Professor of Psychology in the Yale University Department of Psychiatry. He is the Past President of the National Association for Drama Therapy, and the Chairperson of the National Coalition of Arts Therapy Associations (NCATA).

Dr. Johnson is the Editor-in-Chief of the *International Journal of Arts in Psychotherapy* and a frequent contributor to many professional journals.

Dr. Johnson majored in drama and psychology as an undergraduate at Yale University. He received his doctorate from the Yale Department of Psychology.

Photographs by **VIRGINIA BLAISDELL,** Art Director of a community newspaper, *The New Haven Independent*. She is also a freelance photographer, and has exhibited widely. She has been photographing the authors' work for ten years.

Waiting at the Gate: Creativity and Hope in the Nursing Home

Activities, Adaptation & Aging
Volume 9, Number 3

CONTENTS

Preface

I dwell in Possibility,
A fairer house than Prose,
More numerous of windows,
Superior for doors.

With chambers, as the cedars,
Impregnable of eye,
And for an everlasting roof,
The gables of the sky.

Of visitors—the fairest—
For occupation—this:
The spreading wide my *eager* hands
To gather Paradise.

As our great-uncle Read finished reciting Emily Dickinson's poem, from memory, he looked out over the Hudson River with quiet serenity. How many times had he read that poem! We were in his Riverside Drive apartment, where he had lived for 45 years, having travelled from Connecticut to talk with him about his life and memories of the family. He was 95 years old. He had begrudgingly permitted us to interview him on videotape, his interest in preserving family history outweighing his suspicions that we thought he might be getting old.

"Now I want you to look at the last line! . . . What does it say?" We looked down at the open book we had tried to hand him, which he had tossed back as if insulted.

"It says, 'The spreading wide my narrow hands.'"

"That's right! You noticed I used *eager*."

"Yes."

"I thought I could improve on Emily."

The creative spark, active mind, and lifelong dedication to the vision of a worldwide community kept the light kindled in this man's mind until his body gave up, in mid-sentence, two years later. "Keep everything open," he often exhorted us. That's why he didn't have curtains on his windows: they blocked the view. He is an inspiration for our work, and serves as a constant reminder that nurturing one's creativity keeps the soul vital.

This book reflects a decade of our work creating "possibility" in nursing homes; of keeping individuals as well as the institution open instead of closed. In 1976 we found ourselves interested in learning more about the elderly. As activity therapists at the Yale Psychiatric Institute, a long-term psychiatric hospital, we had witnessed the power of the therapeutic community in helping severely disturbed people and the important role the creative arts therapies played in enriching that experience. So the nursing home was an easy transition for us. Here was a long-term residential setting with the potential for becoming a therapeutic community. We were challenged by the vision of transforming the psychosocial environment of the nursing home into the healing community we had so carefully and lovingly developed in the psychiatric setting.

There were many reasons why we made this transition. Perhaps one of the most important, though we were unaware of it at the time, was the loss of our grandparents. By 1979 all had died. Both of us had significant attachments to our grandparents; in our relationships with our elderly patients we rediscovered our roles as grandchildren and found a new source of solace.

We began by offering weekly movement and drama therapy groups at the Sound View Specialized Care Center in West Haven, Connecticut, a 100-bed skilled nursing facility. Over the years, our involvement there increased, and we provided a wide range of therapeutic activities in the creative arts. Susan became the Coordinator of Psychosocial Programs, and David began consulting in other nursing homes. A few years later, Susan became the Administrator of the New Haven Convalescent Center, and David became the head of a geropsychology training program on the Nursing Home Care Unit at the Veteran's Administration Hospital. We were now in administrative and training positions, and began to learn about the complexities of long-term care from a larger perspective, while attempting to understand how the creative arts therapies could contribute to the overall mission of the facility.

As the intergenerational program between the New Haven Convalescent Center and the neighboring Barnard Elementary School developed, both of us participated in the planning of large-scale artistic rituals in which these and many other facilities joined together in sharing their creativity and life. We discovered that the creative arts not only contribute to the health and hopefulness of an individual, not only bring a sense of intimacy, sharing, and esteem to a small group of elderly, but also impact powerfully on large communities of people, some of whom may be institutionalized, and some of whom may live normal lives in the community.

Many of these chapters have been published in journals as separate articles and could be read in any order. Nevertheless, we have placed them in a sequence that illustrates the progression in our understanding from basic concepts and methods to more sophisticated ideas. We think that the reader's appreciation of the later chapters will be substantially enhanced if the earlier ones have been read first. The section, "Healing Elements in Movement and Drama Therapy," presents our basic model and conceptualization of therapeutic process, including chapters on the basic methods and healing elements of movement and drama therapy. The second section, "Explorations in the Therapeutic Process," examines specific concepts such as reminiscence, sexuality, and transference, and describes techniques that we have found useful with the confused. The third section, "The Arts and Communitas," focuses on the impact of the arts therapies on the general atmosphere and communal spirit of the nursing home, through playful intergenerational workshops and community rituals.

While we firmly believe that the creative arts therapies as a whole (including art, dance, drama, music, and poetry) share fundamental links and have similar effects (Johnson, 1985), we have chosen to focus on movement and drama therapy in this book, for these are our special expertise. Yet this book could not have been completed without the inspiration and courage we have gained from our collaboration with many creative arts therapists, whose insight and perseverance in developing a new field will, we know, make significant contributions to the care of the elderly.

We would like to acknowledge the advice, support, and encouragement of Henry Harrison, Dr. Joseph Camilleri, and the Board of Directors of the New Haven Convalescent Center, Dr. Jacob Levine and Anne Anastasio at the V.A, and Dr. Judith Gordon at the University of New Haven. We are grateful for the assistance of our co-authors, Maryellen Kelleher, Betsy Mason-Luckey, and Marilyn B. Margolis. Most importantly, we are indebted to our patients who over these past ten years have taught us, challenged us, and shared themselves so openly and with so much wisdom and courage. You have given us many gifts; perhaps, with this book, we can offer something in return.

Susan L. Sandel
David Read Johnson

Introduction

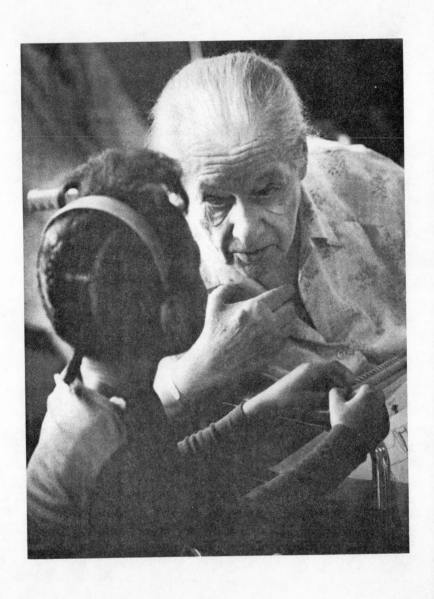

Chapter One
Creativity and Hope in the Nursing Home: An Emerging Vision

Susan L. Sandel
David Read Johnson

I WANTED THIS,
I WISHED FOR THAT,
THERE'S NO POINT TO WANT
FOR THERE I SAT.

WAIT,
WAIT,
WAIT BY THE GATE.
PRETTY SOON
YOU'LL KNOW YOUR FATE.

The refrain sung by the group of nursing home residents in a movement-drama therapy session filled the room with energy and laughter, for waiting is both a well-known friend and foe to them. The "gate" refers to the nurses' station, where those who are able line up in their wheelchairs in order to make requests or demands. The poem developed into a role-play:

Sadie: I need help with my food; can't you see it's getting cold!
Arthur: That's nothing. I need a bedpan. Soon.
Jules: Please, we've been waiting so long!
The NURSE, played by Louise, covered her eyes and shrunk her body as far as she could into her chair, apparently trying to disappear.
Sadie: She dried up.

Jules: We used her up.
Arthur: Now what will we do?

Louise: Wait by the gate!

Waiting is a reality of institutional life that must be acknowledged. Even in the best nursing home, with a dedicated staff and aesthetically pleasing environment, people must wait to have some of their most basic needs met. Waiting to be taken to an activity; waiting for a bedpan, and then to be cleaned up; waiting for relatives to visit; waiting to be fed. A waiting that expresses one's lack of control, one's complete dependency on someone else, that is grounded in one's disability and fuels one's sense of weakness. The anger, even outrage, generated by this condition is tempered, however, by the fear that there will not be enough help, enough staff, enough energy to fulfill one's needs. And so one waits, and doesn't complain.

In addition to the waiting related to dependency, there is the waiting created by not having anything meaningful to do, of having disengaged from the practical world: the people lined up along the hall, who are *just there*. To the infrequent visitor of the nursing home it is this image of passivity, of emptiness, that haunts the soul and cries out for an explanation, and usually ends in an aversion to the nursing home itself.

Finally, there is the waiting for death. The image is a familiar one: the disoriented elderly person, turned inward in a reverie of memory, waiting patiently for the end. Nursing homes used to be perceived as places where people were sent in order to wait to die. The nursing home of forty years ago was portrayed in this manner by one social activist, Edith Sterns, in an article titled "Buried Alive," (1947):

> Unlike some primitive tribes, we do not kill off our aged and infirm. We bury them alive in institutions. To save our face, we call the institutions homes—a travesty on the word. I have seen dozens of such homes in the last six months—desolate places peopled with blank-faced men and women, one home so like the other that each visit seemed a recurrent nightmare.

Dr. Robert Butler, in his Pulitzer Prize winning book, *Why Survive? Being Old in America* (1975), which stirred our country to a new consciousness about ageism, referred to the typical nursing home as a "house of death" where the old were warehoused. Butler also shared his vision of the new kind of nursing home that would be a growth-promoting environment for both the residents and the community:

> A nursing home should not be exclusively oriented to the care of its inpatients but rather should supply services beyond its walls. It should be the hub of many activities. . . There should be a social and intellectual climate that makes it possible for the elderly who can and wish to do so to study, grow, and enjoy themselves. There should be a freedom of action and a sense of community. Individual identity and dignity can be maintained through social contact, the presence of familiar possessions, and the exercise of personal freedom and choice (p. 295).

Butler's words heralded a revolution in nursing homes during the past ten years. Public awareness about the increasing numbers of old-old Americans, the psychosocial needs of the aged and their families, and the ongoing dilemma of health care costs has catapulted us into a health care revolution that is still in tumult and transition. The new vision has generated higher standards and expectations in our consumer-conscious society. The downward path of expectations that formerly equated nursing homes with stagnation and death is being replaced with a new view that demands the preservation of human dignity and vitality. Novelist Robert Oliphant (1985) writes,

> Today our expectations [of nursing homes] are much higher. We expect nursing homes to do much more than provide custodial care for a few neglected old people. Rather, we expect them to take the place of the family, to take the place of society in providing a safe, hospitable environment, to offer social and rehabilitation programs, and to accommodate a clientele that grows older and more numerous each year (p. 20).

A new language is emerging: life-cycle psychology, continuum of care, life-care communities and campuses. The death terminology associated with long-term care is being replaced with a life-cycle orientation and language that now encompasses a life span of 20-30 years after retirement. "Houses of death" are becoming "houses of life," ranging from retirement communities to life-care campuses that have accomodations ranging from apartments to skilled nursing facilities. A growing emphasis on "quality of life" in all types of long-term care has precipitated an interest in recreational, social, cultural and religious activities for the aged. Family members and health-care professionals looking for nursing homes and related facilities exhibit a more sophisticated level of awareness concerning therapeutic activities programs and the daily recreational activity routine. In a recent nationwide survey of nursing home residents, activities were cited as the second most significant concern after staff competency and training (Spalding and Frank, 1985.) Dr. Thelma Fogelberg (1985), an 85-year-old nursing home resident, summarized this enlightened view:

> The ideal home is something that everyone from childhood to old age longs for. For the person who resides in a nursing home, the term ideal home has a special meaning. The home must be well-structured, attractive and capable of fulfilling the emotional as well as the physical needs of individuals. It must also sustain the concept of a home as the place for nurturing the growth and development of individual powers of thinking, feeling and being. (p. 52)

The increased expectations of this vision have impacted on all aspects of nursing home care. These include (1) improved medical and physical care, (2) a secure and attractive physical environment, (3) competent administration and staff training, (4) enriching recreational and occupational activities, (5) sophisticated spiritual and psychological services, and (6) substantial contact with families and the surrounding community.

This vision, to make the nursing home a living, creative, and humane environment, is one response to the exposure of the inadequacies of long-term care in this country. An alternative response has been to call for the elimination of nursing homes, through the development of home-based health care, alternative settings, and expansion of specialized hospital programs. This viewpoint often minimizes the problem of long-term care by citing the fact that only 5% of the elderly are living in nursing homes, and by advocating a greater focus on the needs of the "well-elderly," as if the attention nursing homes receive detracts from the needs of the healthy elderly. There are those who would question the assumption that an institutional setting such as a nursing home could *ever* be an enriching environment; that it is best to develop alternative services in our families and communities rather than spend scarce resources in a futile attempt to salvage the nursing home.

We very much believe that the nursing home can become the therapeutic and growth-enhancing community that Butler and others have envisioned. Our experience with therapeutic communities in psychiatric institutions, and with several nursing homes over the past decade has convinced us of the potential value of communal life within creative and stimulating institutions (Almond, 1974). After all, what is a nursing home but a building and people? There is nothing innately and unchangeably horrible about it. Society's fear of the nursing home or psychiatric ward is not based on their being institutions (for most people work every day in institutions), but on people's ignorance and fear of death and disability. An additional influence is the high value placed on individualism in American culture, which views congregate or group-living with suspicion or as inferior to living "on one's own" (Riesman, 1950; Slater, 1970).

We believe these attitudes can change. We have discovered that life in a nursing home, filled with activities, people, and stimulation, can bring meaning, challenge, and happiness to an elderly person who otherwise might be spending his days alone in his house, encased in ever more restrictive ritual and isolation. Just as the adolescent is faced with a number of options in the transition to young adulthood (e.g., to stay at home, go to college or into the service, move out into his own house), so the elderly person is faced with options (e.g., to stay at home, move to an apartment or congregate living center, or into a nursing home). Hopefully these decisions will be based on the rational considerations of convenience, level of care needed, finances, etc., and not confused by a societal prejudice that characterizes the nursing home as an inferior and shameful choice (Boling, 1984). There is no reason why this late age transition cannot also be experienced as a natural one that provides many good alternatives, including moving to a nursing home. One of the major reasons why the nursing home will be a viable option in the future is the contribution to this humane environment that is being made by the creative arts therapies.

THE ROLE OF THE CREATIVE ARTS THERAPIES

The creative arts therapies have played a significant role in the enlivening of long-term care environments and the creation of the new nursing home. Activities that foster passive participation, such as movies, entertainments, and events for which the elderly are the audience, i.e., passive recipients of pleasurable stimuli, are consistent with the "waiting to die" assumption of the old nursing home. Active participation in stimulating and creative experiences with the goals of involvement, expression, and interaction has become more valued in the new nursing home of the 1980's. The philosophy, techniques and approaches of the creative arts therapies have been incorporated into the training of activities/recreation personnel and pervade reports in professional and trade journals concerned with aging. In some states, the role of the creative arts therapist has been formally recognized in designated job lines, or at least recognized as an alternative to more traditional recreation training for nursing home personnel.

This book is about the contributions of the creative arts therapies, specifically movement and drama therapy, to the individual and communal welfare of residents in nursing homes. The arts provide structured interpersonal events in which self-esteem, personal achievement, interaction, and expression are enhanced. The arts are symbolic and abstract, and at the same time concrete and visceral. Like crafts, sports, games, and parties, they involve action in the real world with other people. However, the arts also give access to the inner life of feeling, dream, and imagination. In this way they are similar to introspection, prayer, and psychotherapy. The arts are thus means by which the inner life becomes manifest: this is their unique power and the source of their potential contribution (McNiff, 1981; Robbins, 1980).

The chapters in this book will describe the various ways that movement and drama therapy impact on the health of the elderly person. We believe they contribute in five major areas:

1. *Increasing orientation and activation:* The creative arts therapies provide a structured interpersonal environment in which organized sensory stimulation, simplified interpersonal interaction, and physical action facilitate orientation, attention, and arousal.
2. *Facilitating reminiscence:* By providing concrete physical and

imaginative cues through sound, touch, play and visual forms, the creative arts therapies enhance the process of reminiscence by facilitating access to deeper memories, as well as the subsequent sharing of these memories with others in a group context.

3. *Increasing self-understanding and acceptance:* By encouraging spontaneous expression through the arts media, aspects of the self that have been kept from awareness often emerge. Work in these media usually increases the person's curiosity about him/herself, and with the help of a therapist or other members of the group, the person can discover the unique meanings of these self-expressions, and learn to accept him/herself for his limitations as well as his strengths.

4. *Developing meaningful interpersonal relationships:* The creative arts therapies provide a means of structured communication among people. A setting of intimacy is created through the mutual expression of aspects of their inner lives. Yet, due to the concrete, nonverbal nature of the arts media, people with cognitive or language deficits can participate equally. The atmosphere of play, fun, and spontaneity contributes to the bonding among members of the group.

5. *Building communal spirit:* Communal artistic events such as murals, songs, performances, celebrations, or workshops have tremendous power to link people of divergent backgrounds, cultures, ages, or conditions, and to articulate their common bond with the institution. The arts support a sense of belonging that expresses the inner vision of its participants. Thus, the creative arts therapies can make a major contribution to intergenerational programs, or to events linking the nursing home to its wider community and to other institutions.

Participation in creative arts therapies is an antidote to the dependency, passivity, and death that waiting expresses. The creative arts therapies envision the client as an artist, a creator of his own self and life. The artwork, whether it be a painting, song, or dance, directly symbolizes the self-in-the-world, and represents autonomy, activity, and life. The creative moment begins when the aging nursing home resident, as artist, confronts the representation of the void: the blank page, the empty canvas, the moment of silence. In creating the sound or movement or shape, the person has the opportunity to recapture elements of the self-in-the-past and to create new images of self-in-the-present. For what fills the page or canvas or silence is not a design, a plan, or prearranged model, but rather the spontaneous expression of one's insides. In filling the canvas, the artist deals with the void, with death, and seeks another answer to "What is the point?" Susanne Langer (1953) said that the pleasure of beauty is the perception of a life wholly significant. The creative arts therapies offer a way toward a life of significance, otherwise so threatened by custodial care. Successful artistic expression is powerful because it reassures us that significance and meaning can emerge out of nothing. As these qualities are revealed in creative activity, the perceptions of both the elderly person and those around him are affected. Seeing elderly people moving, making music, or enacting a drama instills feelings of hope and affirms their humanness, no matter how limited their abilities.

So the creative arts therapies facilitate the preservation of life, of meaning, and of hope, by seeking the beautiful and playful aspects of the self, and valuing humor, flexibility, and spontaneity in relationships with others. These values challenge the "waiting to die" phenomenon of the custodial nursing home, and offer lively alternatives to the resident in the new institution of the 1990's.

I. Healing Elements of Movement and Drama Therapy

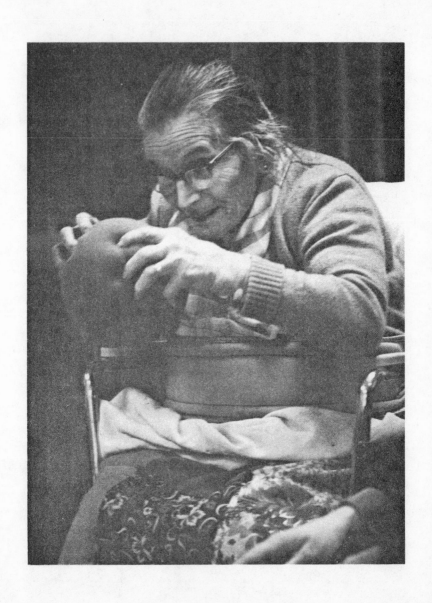

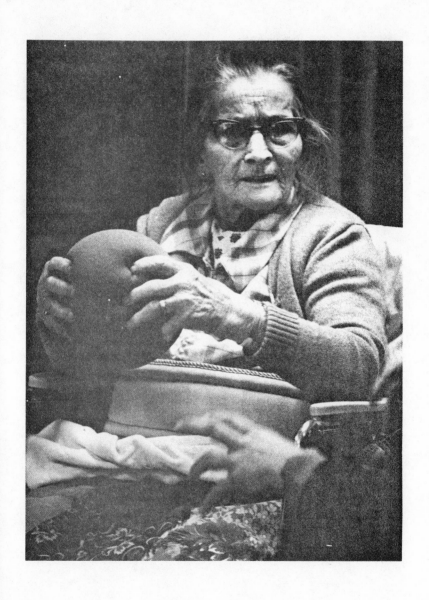

Chapter Two
Principles of Group Treatment in a Nursing Home

David Read Johnson
Susan L. Sandel
Marilyn B. Margolis

The increasing focus in recent years on institutional care for the elderly has brought psychosocial and recreation programming in nursing homes under greater scrutiny. A 1976 Survey of Institutionalized Persons conducted by the Bureau of Census revealed that nursing home residents were least satisfied with activity programs compared to other aspects of institutional life (Cook, 1981). Many programs apparently do not meet the wide range of patient needs, although a consensus on what their rationales should be has not emerged.

One rationale for activities programs has been to make the patients feel comfortable and happy. Activities in which patients remain passive recipients of pleasurable stimuli, such as parties, films and entertainments, characterize many long-term care programs. Another rationale stresses the importance of maintaining patients' interests in previously acquired skills and has led to programs involving arts and crafts. These programs emphasize the patient's relationship to the skill and the product.

A third rationale emphasizes the development of meaningful interpersonal relationships and offers programs in which social interaction among patients and staff is the central focus. However, programs of this type may conflict with the atmosphere of disengagement in many nursing homes where social interactions among distressed or confused patients are a source of stress for personnel. Activities that focus on social interaction usually involve the most

Originally published in the *Journal of Long-Term Care Administration*, Winter, 1982, 19-24. Reprinted by permission of the American College of Health Care Administrators.

alert, verbally responsive patients. Confused or disturbed people are typically unable to participate in such programming because of their disruptive behavior. The lack of training of recreation and administrative personnel in various forms of psychosocial treatment, particularly in approaches which are appropriate for less alert and less verbal patients, contributes to the slow development of more sophisticated milieus in nursing homes (Butler, 1981).

An opportunity now exists to apply principles of group, milieu, and activity therapies which have been developed for 30 years in psychiatric settings to long-term care for the elderly. A sophisticated body of knowledge about this work is available for nursing home administrators and personnel to draw upon and to adapt to their own settings (Almond, 1974; Cummings & Cummings, 1962; Edelson, 1970; Jones, 1953). These approaches to the treatment of confused, disturbed, and incarcerated people provide a rich framework for creating group programs in long-term care facilities.

The authors initially created a psychosocial milieu program at the Sound View Specialized Care Center based upon group and activity therapy principles developed in psychiatric therapeutic communities (Mosey, 1973; Sandel, 1980; Johnson, 1981a). Sound View is a 100-bed skilled nursing facility which treats both short-term patients for intensive rehabilitation and a smaller population of long-term geriatric patients. The program began ten years ago with the introduction of two movement therapy groups. The core program consisted of recreational and group therapy activities, including movement therapy, drama therapy, a discussion group for male patients, poetry and music groups, and a special group program for confused patients. Parties, crafts, visiting entertainers, and games were also provided. Nursing, physical therapy, and social work staff participated with recreation and group therapy staff, aided by volunteers and student interns from nearby colleges. Psychosocial programs were actively supported by the administrative staff, who coordinated the integration of these programs with social services and nursing care.

Most of the groups met weekly for one hour and consisted of six to twelve patients. Patient membership in the groups was consistent from week to week. Patients' levels of cognitive functioning, alertness, and verbal facility seemed to be the critical factors for referral to particular groups, rather than the severity of their physical disabilities. Thus, there was a wide range of physical functioning among members of each group.

The program's guiding principle has been that patients can benefit from meaningful interpersonal relationships which are nurtured through activity and engagement. Patients in nursing homes have been removed from the family network of relationships, either because the family has been unable to care for the patient or because there is no more family. The task of creating a meaningful social network now lies within the milieu of the nursing home where the person may spend several years.

The creation of an atmosphere of engagement and meaningful interpersonal relations may be accomplished through three means. First, group leaders establish a stable and safe environment in the group, one well-protected and consistent, so that a clear group identity can be formed. Second, the sharing of reminiscences which are stimulated by the group activities is encouraged. In this way, linkages among members are forged from similarities of experiences and empathetic responses to each other's struggles. Third, a gradual shift to here-and-now interactions among participants is facilitated by supportive confrontation of people's physical and mental limitations, approaching deaths, and other important life events.

We will now describe these three principles of intervention in greater detail.

ESTABLISHING A STABLE ENVIRONMENT

A prerequisite for meaningful interpersonal relationships is the establishment of a safe and familiar environment. For confused patients, consistency of time, location, and group membership can be important orienting cues. We have found that patients are able to associate a group with a particular day or room and will then remember why they have been brought together. One patient, for example, was completely disoriented while alone in his bedroom and even while being wheeled down the hall. However, as soon as he entered the activities room where the same people were doing the same thing, he said, "Well, I'm here in the drama group—it must be Thursday!" He and other patients used this consistent weekly event to locate other events: "Yesterday I went to the drama group, so today must be Friday."

The creation of a consistent, orienting environment is greatly facilitated by bodily activity. Movement helps to concretize interpersonal events and brings greater organization to patients' responses (Johnson, 1982a). In our psychosocial programs, consistency is maintained in the group's activities. Beginning and ending each session with a group ritual, such as holding hands and making a sound or cheer, serves as a reliable indicator of where we are and who we are. Patients' abilities to predict and recognize these repetitive events support their feelings of control and stability. The group provides a concrete and relatively simple structure for social interaction. As patients' investments and use of these group rituals increase, the need for idiosyncratic, personal rituals (e.g., hair pulling) often decreases in response to the anxiety-lowering effects of the group environment. For example, one woman quickly gave up her continual complaining in order to participate in the repetitive movement and sound exercises of the movement therapy group.

We mobilize a group identity from a consistent and well-bounded group. Each group gives itself a name which the participants chant in unison at the end of the meeting. Signs on the door listing the names and meeting times of each group serve as a reminder to everyone that the groups occur regularly. Developing consistent interactions with each patient, such as reminding them of our names, saying hello to each in the beginning of the session, and using our personal energy to become a central figure in the group environment, allows them to identify the leaders with the group. We emerge as forceful and trustworthy presences in the group, and are often identified and remembered by confused patients. The development and maintenance of a stable social and physical environment not only produces a trusting atmosphere, but also seems necessary in order for many patients to develop a consistent image or memory of the group experience.

Soon after the development of a group identity and differentiation of the therapist/leader as a symbol of the group, individual members begin to develop identifiable roles. These roles support their sense of self, and are often associated with particular group activities. In one movement therapy group the beginning ritual consisted of each member, in turn, leading the group with a simple movement and sound. Anna, an 86-year old woman, always did the same thing. Every time, she extended her arms toward the center of the circle, saying "ahhh" softly. When she was transferred to another nursing home, the therapist asked if people remembered Anna. They did not, until one woman opened her arms and said "ahhh" just as Anna had done. The whole group responded with recognition and jointly performed this movement and sound. We believe that this level of orientation cannot occur without the establishment of a safe and consistent group atmosphere.

SHARED REMINISCENCE

Reminiscing is used as a vehicle for sharing and communicating with others about meaningful relationships; therefore, the focus is on the quality of the interpersonal interactions more than on each individual's personal integration of past experiences (Butler, 1974). Until the group creates its own repertoire of mutual experiences, people's pasts are the richest source of meaningful interaction. One goal is to facilitate the communal sharing of these experiences so that linkages among group members can occur.

Concrete physical activities are useful in stimulating associations to past experiences with significant others. The use of unison activity provides a structure for sharing reminiscences about similar experiences. The activity stimulates associations and images which can be used to facilitate patients' verbalization of their memories.

In one movement therapy group the participants were all stretching their arms toward the center of the circle and pulling them back to their chests, while making rhythmic sounds. The therapist asked, "What could we pull?" One man answered, "A rope on a boat." "We're rowing!" exclaimed another patient. The therapist then asked, "Where are we rowing? Who is with us? What river are we on?" and other questions that elicited specific memories from group members who were then encouraged to share their responses in more detail. One woman remembered a river near her childhood home. Another wanted to row home to her son. A man remembered that he had last been on a row boat with his wife the day before they found out she had cancer.

Maintaining the physical activity throughout the verbal reminiscing helps to keep a concrete central focus for the group. As memories are detailed, movements and images may change. For example, this group shifted to memories of fishing, then cooking the fish, then dinner times, and so on. The therapist facilitated the flow of images and associated movements.

In the drama therapy group, images may lead to a role play between two or more people who reenact the scene. Other people then role play similar situations, which often stimulates a lively discussion about their pasts. The role playing, like the movement, serves to link these past memories to current interactions among group members.

As the group identity becomes established and social interaction increases, the participants are more successful in calling up and sharing memories about their lives. Initially, idiosyncratic memories may be mentioned out of context of the group's discussion or activity. However, soon the process of shared reminiscence leads participants to learn about each other. Often group members become associated with significant people of the past. For example, the therapist becomes linked with the patient's children, or a male patient is identified with someone's husband. Stimulating such associations supports the transfer of significance from past to current relationships. In this way, shared reminiscence serves an important function as a stepping stone to here-and-now relationships.

MEANINGFUL GROUP INTERACTION

One of the major obstacles to meaningful group interaction is the reality of the patients' situations. Many of the people we work with are in wheelchairs and have severe and multiple handicaps, including hearing or visual impairments, strokes, amputations, aphasia, and incontinence. Many experience severe memory loss or other cognitive deficits. Some are approaching death. Most have lost their spouse and other loved ones. As group identity and trust develop, these painful realities become harder for participants to ignore. Moving their bodies, raising their voices, and reminiscing evoke people's feelings about their losses, declining health, and remaining hopes. We have observed that sometimes patients feel stupid, incompetent, or humiliated when they cannot do a movement or speak "well." Some are able to express their jealousy of the youth, "wholeness," and enthusiasm of the therapists. Many are afraid that their physical deterioration will be ridiculed or that they will be rejected by the group. Some may complain about "those old ugly people." We began to understand why for some people disorientation might be preferable to the depressing reality of their situation. One 96-year old woman often cried out, "Please, please, only pleasant things! Let's talk about pleasant things!"

Our initial timidity in confronting patients' limitations and concerns began to have negative effects on the groups. Once each group demonstrated its trust in us, our uncomfortable avoidance of difficult issues confirmed for the patients that their problems were indeed embarassing and anxiety-arousing for others. Our denial of painful issues was interpreted by the patients as fear, and inhibited the developing of an atmosphere of spontaneity and open discussion.

Since our strategy had been to create a safe and consistent environment by controlling the groups' boundaries, membership, and activities, we now needed more than ever to be seen as forceful presences ready to protect members from both external and internal threats. Not only did we prevent intruders from interrupting the groups, we were also quick to confront aggressive participants whose behavior might be intimidating to others.

As this sense of control became established, we no longer avoided dealing with people's problems. Instead of altering an exercise so that a particular patient might not confront his or her disability, we encouraged the group to help the person find a way to adapt to the exercise. Maintaining the regular activities of the session and identifying difficulties seem to allow patients to talk openly about the feelings they were experiencing. For example, a patient named Michael had a stroke which resulted in the paralysis of his left arm. He often needed to use a brace. In our groups people commonly held hands in a circle. Often another patient showed anxiety or hesitation in reaching out and holding Michael's disabled hand; he, too, balked at offering it.

> *Therapist*: You can hold Michael's hand, Evelyn.
> *Evelyn*: I don't want to hurt it.
> *Therapist*: Michael has had a stroke and doesn't have full use of his hand, but you won't hurt it.
> *Michael*: Here it is. Pretty bad excuse for a hand.
> *Therapist*: You seem ashamed of it, Michael.
> *Michael*: It's no damned good.
> *Evelyn*: Like my legs.
> *Therapist*: You feel bad about the things that don't work so well, don't you?
> *Michael*: Yes, it makes me mad too.
> *Therapist*: Yes, how about other people? (Other people talk about their physical problems.)
> *Therapist*: Evelyn, you've got Michael's hand. How does it feel?
> *Evelyn*: Nice and warm.
> *Therapist*: Good. Let's continue our exercise, okay?

In a similar manner, loss of spouses and the inevitability of death were also able to be addressed. With each discussion, the group members became more tolerant of these subjects, and appeared less anxious during the day (Benaim, 1957).

One drama therapy group that had attained this level of intimacy was able to discuss a variety of distressing subjects. In one session, they had been given pretzels which had been cooked in another recreation activity. They did not like them.

Linda: They're not real pretzels.

Cecilia: Not very good.

John: (who is a reverend): A first class flop! (General agreement and laughter among everyone.)

(The therapist leads a chant of "first class flop" accompanied by arm movements directed toward the center of the circle where the pretzel has been placed.)

Cecilia: I think we've hurt its feelings.

Linda: Throw it away! Go on, Reverend, say something.

John: (smiling): Ashes to ashes. (Laughter.)

Therapist: This is like a burial.

Audrey: Yes. I think we should bury it. (Therapist leads the group in a mock burial of the pretzels.)

John: And may we never see *you* again! (aggressively)

Therapist: It's as if we've buried a person. How would people feel after *you* died?

Sally: They probably would say good riddance.

John: When you're gone, the others just have to go on living.

Audrey: I'm a burden on them—they'd like to see us go; you can tell that sometimes. They're too polite to say it.

Cecilia: They'll never say it. (General discussion about family members who visit and pretend all is well.)

Therapist: That must hurt.

Sally: I feel like a bag of nothing. They might as well just throw me away. (Silence follows.)

Audrey: I feel like that sometimes too. Oh well.

John: *We'll* remember you. They will too.

Linda: Who made that pretzel anyway?

Therapist: Alice (a staff member). Are you going to tell her about it?

Sally: Oh no!

Audrey: It would hurt her feelings.

Cecilia: Such a nice girl.

In this process, the therapist is a supportive guide for patients who are struggling to face their life situations. The therapist does not indiscriminately bring up distressing subjects, "forcing" patients to deal with their problems. This would be provocative and could be experienced by patients as an attack. The atmosphere of safety would be shattered. The goal is always to create a culture of tolerance and spontaneity in which meaningful contact among people is encouraged.

CONCLUSION

Our psychosocial group programs stress the values of activity, engagement, and interpersonal relationships. They are based on the concept of a therapeutic community. Positive changes in patients' orientation, clinical state, and satisfaction have been observed as a result of these programs in various settings.

The fact that many geriatric patients who are approaching death naturally begin to disengage from their social milieu is not a reason to structure the institution in a way which insists on disengagement. As our patients' health deteriorates, they do begin to disengage from their groups. We do not prevent this. Rather, we encourage each group to recognize this process, and have found that everyone benefits as they find ways to say goodbye to a disengaging member. The fact that the group cares and remembers people is very reassuring to those whose separation is imminent. The group, like the family, will go on. Our groups often have anniversary parties in which the participants review the history of the group and mention former members.

The formation of groups which tolerate meaningful relationships among patients takes time, energy, and support from nursing and administrative personnel. Bringing people together in these kinds of groups mobilizes all the complexity, distress, and rewards of human interactions. The potential for disruption is great in settings where social interactions among confused or distressed patients have been sources of staff stress. Staff training and enlightened administration are crucial for such a program and its values to be integrated into the institution.

Forty years ago psychiatric institutions were like many of today's nursing homes: recreation programs provided crafts or passive entertainment, patients had no formal meetings with each other, and treatment was administered by a doctor or nurse to each isolated individual. Psychiatric treatment has been revolutionized by attempts to utilize the therapeutic aspects of the patients' social milieu.

The introduction of appropriately adapted and well administered psychosocial treatment approaches into nursing home care could significantly improve the quality of life among the institutionalized elderly.

Chapter Three
A Psychosocial Approach to Dance-Movement Therapy

Susan L. Sandel
Maryellen Kelleher

In our mechanized society, with its emphasis on leisure time, people become less and less active with advancing age. This is often encouraged by well-meaning friends and relatives, who urge the elderly to take it easy and not to strain themselves when participating in sports or performing household chores. For those confined to a convalescent home these problems are intensified. There, the older person's role is typically that of a passive recipient of nursing care. Often the staff is too busy providing basic medical care to focus on the residents' other physical and psychosocial needs. An atmosphere in which motionlessness prevails is not unusual in many nursing homes. The severely restricted capabilities of the patients themselves and the confining nature of the institution tend to reinforce this inactivity.

INACTIVITY AND AGING

Many disabilities commonly associated with old age are accepted as an inevitable consequence of growing old. Recently, researchers and clinicians have begun to challenge this longstanding belief. They are learning that many of the health problems of older people are not the inevitable consequence of old age but the result of a sedentary life style (Bortz, 1981; deVries, 1974; Kraus, 1956).

For example, one of the most common conditions of old age, arteriosclerosis, is characterized by accumulation of fatty deposits in

Originally published as "'Dance/Movement Therapy'' (Chapter 8), in *Physical Fitness and the Older Person* (1984), edited by Leonard Biegel. Copyright 1984. Reprinted by permission of Aspen Publishers, Inc.

the arteries of the heart, brain, extremities, and kidneys. Arterio-sclerosis contributes to heart disease, stroke, walking disabilities, and poor organ function and accounts for approximately half of all deaths in the United States. Commonly thought to be an inevitable consequence of old age, arteriosclerosis is actually the result of de-creased activity (Keelor, 1976). As one ages and becomes less ac-tive, muscle mass is replaced by fat tissue. Conversely, increasing the amount of muscle mass can help to counteract fatty tissue replacement; muscle mass can be increased, regardless of age, through physical activity.

Inactivity also contributes to a host of other symptoms associated with old age. Inactivity facilitates accumulation of free-floating ten-sion, manifested in such symptoms as insomnia, irritableness, and restlessness (Gulton, 1975). This is especially so for those confined to bed or wheelchair, who get very little exercise. Restlessness and insomnia are often treated with drug therapy or physical restraint rather than with activities designed to reduce tension.

Depression is another condition prevalent among the institutional-ized elderly. Loss of societal role, material deprivation, physical de-cline, or loss of a spouse can trigger depression. One of the prime signs of depression is inactivity. A vicious cycle can easily develop in which depression and inactivity reinforce each other, and it can become increasingly difficult for the individual to interrupt this de-bilitating pattern.

Physical activity stimulates functioning of the respiratory, circu-latory, and skeletal systems. Exercise also promotes and maintains muscle tone, balance and coordination, and spatial orientation. The old adage, "use it or lose it," applies not only to physical vigor, but to memory, orientation, social skills, and the ability to give and receive affection.

TREATMENT MODALITIES

Movement is a part of many different treatment modalities for the aged. Physical therapy (including exercise programs) as well as cre-ative movement and dance/movement therapy all utilize physical ac-tivity. Fitness programs offer exercises of varying levels of difficulty, depending upon the stamina and overall health of the participants. Goals of such programs might include increased mobility, improved circulation and breathing, and relaxation and release of tension;

emotional well-being is a byproduct of better physical functioning. Although exercise programs are usually performed in a group, the emphasis is on the individual's experience and improvement.

Dance Movement Therapy

Creative movement, as a therapy for the aged, has been widely used in nursing homes and senior centers recently. Goals of creative movement programs include the same ones that characterize fitness programs (with the additional aims of increasing self-esteem and social interaction) (Herman & Renzurri, 1978). Classes include a variety of movement activities, often accompanied by music, designed to encourage creativity, spontaneity, and bodily awareness within a social setting.

Dance/movement therapy integrates physiological, psychological, and sociological aspects and attemps to give meaning to movement through the development of images within the movement interaction. While encouraging emotional reactions and processing of affective responses (both positive and negative), dance/movement therapy also facilitates social interaction. Movement activities are not the goal of the group experience, but rather the tool for creating a therapeutic environment. This approach distinguishes dance/movement therapy from other physical movement therapies and offers a comprehensive treatment method for the elderly.

Dance/Movement Distinctions

The American Dance Therapy Association defines dance/movement therapy as '' the psychotherapeutic use of movement as a process which furthers the emotional and physical integration of the individual.'' It is distinguished from other uses of dance (i.e., purely social) by its focus on the nonverbal communicative aspects of behavior and the use of movement as the mode of intervention in the therapeutic relationship. Dance/movement therapy includes a variety of approaches in which the therapist and client use movement as a medium for communication (Chaiklin & Schmais, 1975). Approaches usually do not rely on structured exercises but rather on the spontaneous unfolding of interaction among participants.

Presently, the terms "dance" and "movement" therapy are used interchangeably. Although the American Dance Therapy Association recognizes a Registered Dance Therapist as the qualified practitioner, "movement" is used by therapists who wish to convey a broader meaning to their work. Particularly in geriatric settings, the term movement therapy is more widely used because "dance" is easily misunderstood by people who feel that their physical capabilities are limited. Even the term movement therapy may require explanation, because it can be confused with physical or occupational therapy.

History of Dance/Movement Therapy

Dance/movement therapy was introduced into geriatric patient programs as early as 1942, when Marian Chace, a pioneer of group dance therapy for hospitalized psychiatric patients, began working with elderly patients at St. Elizabeth's Hospital in Washington, D.C. Since then, several therapists have been refining and adapting dance/movement therapy techniques for use with convalescent home patients (Fersh, 1980; Garnet, 1972; Samuels, 1973). The model program created by senior author Susan L. Sandel at the Sound View Specialized Care Center, West Haven, Connecticut, utilizes a group-oriented, interactional approach focusing on the psychosocial benefits to the participants. Action is a vehicle for interaction; physical movement is used to foster social interaction and expression of feelings. Patients also derive physiological benefits from the activity, including improvement in cognitive functioning, which, in turn, affects the ability to interact with others.

Dance/movement therapy seems to have the potential for reaching a wide range of people. Whereas other movement approaches may require task completion, exercise mastery, fine motor coordination, or mental alertness, dance/movement therapy in its most basic form requires participation on a sensory-motor level, thereby tapping into the natural response to rhythm and touch. Patients who might otherwise be excluded from activities can function in a dance/movement therapy group.

Dance/Movement Therapy Techniques

A typical session begins with the patients sitting in a circle (in many convalescent homes, the majority of patients are in wheelchairs). Basic warm-up exercises, which the patients themselves may direct, help to stimulate muscles and nerves. Music initially provides a rhythmic framework, although it need not be used for the entire session. The warm-up movements suggest images that may be related to past life experiences or current concerns. The images provide a focus for meaningful interaction among group members and often stimulate discussion. Sessions always end with a sound and movement ritual that has been created by the group.

Specific techniques that have proved most useful in the authors' model dance/movement therapy program include:

Circle Formation. The circle formation is the primary spatial structure for unison action. It contributes to the feeling of group unity and increases the opportunity for eye contact. Because the therapist and patients are visible to everyone, those with hearing difficulties may participate in group movements by following others. Patients with visual impairments may be seated next to the therapist or other patients, who can describe the activity to them. Although ambulatory participants may move into other spatial formations such as lines, spirals, or a scatter around the room, the circle is still desirable for beginning and ending groups. The circle is particularly desirable for physically disabled and disoriented patients, for it facilitates touch and communication.

Mutual Touch. Mutual touch (such as patting, holding hands, and massage) is an extremely important element of dance/movement therapy sessions. This type of touching differs from the passive touch that convalescent home patients experience when they are bathed, fed, and dressed. Instead of being the passive recipient of physical contact, patients are encouraged to reach out to others to hold hands or pat someone's shoulder. In order to promote an atmosphere of mutuality, the therapist does not manipulate patients' limbs when they are having difficulty performing the movements. The attitude that patients "participate at their own level" is consistent with a nonmanipulative approach.

Music. Music often provides a useful stimulus for beginning a session, because it taps into the natural inclination to respond to rhythm. Music with a clear rhythmic beat is the most useful kind for dance/movement therapy sessions. This can include older music (from the patients' past) or more current music. Music should be playing as the group warms up; however, when recorded or instrumental music interferes with patients making their own sounds, singing songs, or engaging in discussion, the music should be discontinued. The therapist, if seated near the phonograph or tape recorder controls, can fade the music in and out as desired.

Vocalization. Whenever possible, patients should make sounds while moving. Sounding, even a "hum" or an "ah," stimulates breathing, circulation, and central body involvement. This technique is particularly useful for stroke or severely disabled patients whose speech is impaired; they may participate in making group sounds even if they cannot form words or participate in a variety of actions. Any sound that a patient offers is accepted and incorporated into the group experience. As people become more comfortable with vocalization, the therapist might encourage sounds that are expressive of particular feelings by asking, "What kind of sounds do we make when we're happy? sad? angry?" This, in combination with movements, can increase the range of expressive and communicative behavior.

Props. Certain objects are particularly useful for stimulating activity and encouraging interaction among convalescent home patients. Some favorite props are foam "Nerf" balls, colored scarves, and various legnths of stretch material (Lindner et al., 1979). These objects may be used initially to motivate movements such as squeezing, punching, tugging, and throwing, which may develop into participatory games. Props may be used to provide increased sensory stimulation and to link group members together to increase interpersonal awareness.

In groups with disoriented or confused patients, props may be the external focus or support that keeps the group together. In sessions with more alert patients, props may serve as the initial stimuli for interaction but may not be necessary later on (as group members begin to interact freely with one another).

Empathic Movement. One of the major distinguishing characteristics of dance/movement therapy from other body disciplines is the therapist's reliance on empathic movement as the basis for group interaction. Developed by pioneer dance therapist Marian Chace, empathic movement is a technique in which the therapist guides and develops group interaction as it unfolds during the session. Most dance/movement therapists who use this technique do not come to a session with a preconceived plan of activities but rely on verbal and nonverbal cues from the participants, coupled with their own intuitive responses, for the contents of the session. Suggestions, rather than commands, characterize this approach, so that the therapist is cast in the role of catalyst, not teacher.

When using the empathic movement approach, the therapist first creates an atmosphere that encourages self-expression through

movement. The dance/movement therapist then responds to the feelings and thoughts being expressed, rather than imposing specific
muscle movements to condition postural changes or evoke certain
emotions (Chace, 1975). This technique challenges the therapist's
skill in dealing with spontaneous movement expressions and group
process.

Imagery. The development of group images is another technique
of dance/movement therapy distinguishing it from other physical
movement therapies. The use of imagery shifts the experience from
that of a simple action to a symbolic, shared act. A basic guideline
for this technique is to begin with the movement and allow the image
to develop from the action. For example, if the group movement involves stamping feet, the therapist might ask, "What can we stamp
on?" or "Have you ever stamped on something?" This approach
encourages participants to express ideas and associations without
binding the group to the therapist's own imagination.

Imagery can be useful in identifying feelings, relating movements
to real situations, and facilitating reminiscing; thus, the developing
of images gives meaning to the movements. Many patients in convalescent homes are not motivated to exercise for the physical
benefits they might derive. The use of group images switches the
focus from the action to the feelings, thoughts, and memories being
expressed; this provides the motivation for movement.

Reminiscing. Dance/movement therapy sessions with the elderly
provide an opportunity for reminiscing in a social context. Reminiscing by the aged can be an adaptive behavior and should be encouraged in the appropriate circumstances (Butler, 1963; Fallot,
1976; McMahon & Rhudick, 1967). In group dance/movement
therapy, reminiscing may aid in developing interaction among the
participants. For example, rhythmic actions done in unison can un-
cover forgotten memories and feelings. These memories may be
pleasant or painful or of past mastery experiences.

The same guideline that applies to introducing imagery applies
here: always begin with the movement and allow the image (and/or
reminiscence) to develop from the action. Progression from the sensory experience (movement) to a symbolic one (image or association) permits spontaneous unfolding of material during the session.
The therapist need not introduce a topic for the group arbitrarily, but
can pick on the issue or concern suggested by the actual movements
and images.

Benefits to Different Patients

The various goals of dance/movement therapy are appropriate for the needs of most convalescent home patients. Increasing activity, bridging isolation, and encouraging emotional expression and socialization can be helpful to all institutionalized people. Different types of patients within the convalescent home, however, have specific needs, which require variations in therapists' techniques.

Cognitively Impaired. People who suffer from recent memory loss, disorientation, confusion, and other signs of organic brain syndrome can benefit from a consistent and predictable group experience. Consistency in time, place, leadership, and activities helps patients remember or relate to aspects of the group. For example, one very confused woman does not remember the dance/movement therapy session outside of the room where it takes place. Once she enters the room, she knows what to expect and often begins doing warm-up exercises.

Reality orientation techniques may easily be incorporated into the dance/movement therapy session and can be included in the opening and closing rituals. A favorite activity in one of our groups is passing a foam ball and asking participants to say their name when they have the ball. This kind of structured interaction is reassuring when it happens at the beginning of each group; the activity itself becomes an orienting factor for the participants.

When participating in movements that recall past mastery experiences, confused patients often appear more alert and organized. Reminiscing often seems to stimulate immediate, if short-lived, cognitive reorganization.

> One day as I was walking down the hallway gathering people for a group, I heard Ms. B's perseverative wails several doors from her room. The nurse's aide who was attempting to quiet her was relieved when I wheeled Ms. B. to the small room where the group meets. Gradually Ms. B. stopped her wailing, slumped down in her chair, and lapsed into an apparent stupor. "Well," I thought, "at least she's not screaming. Perhaps she feels comfortable here." As group members began their warm-up exercises, which led to reminiscing and conversation, Ms. B. remained unresponsive. Then Mr J. initiated some vigorous swinging arm movements and bell-like sounds. Soon everyone (except Ms. B.) was swinging their arms

rhythmically, chanting "bong, bong, bong." Suddenly Ms. B. lifted her head, opened her eyes, and said "Big Ben." For several minutes she talked lucidly about her travels to London and responded to questions from others. Then her eyes closed and she again lapsed into her sleep-like state for the remainder of the group session.

This kind of experience can change the group's perception of individuals, making it possible to tolerate periodic lapses in their participation or attention.

Physical actions that evoke images of concrete activities such as rowing a boat, washing clothes, or kneading dough usually reawaken memories of past experiences. These provide an excellent vehicle for discussion and sharing even among very confused people.

Direct physical contact also has a dramatic organizing effect on patients who drift in and out of reality. Sometimes people who usually appear disoriented can carry on a lucid conversation when they are holding hands with another person. Movement experiences involving physical contact (holding hands and swaying from side to side or patting other people's hands or faces, for example) are extremely effective in engaging confused patients.

Physically Disabled. Many nursing home patients have severely disabling conditions such as strokes, arthritis, or other degenerative illnesses. Physical limitations need not prevent patients from participating in movement therapy. An accepting, nonjudgmental atmosphere in which people feel free to function within the limits of their own capabilities is most useful for patients with severe physical handicaps. When the focus is on the psychosocial values of the group, rather than on the activity, even the most physically disabled persons can feel that they have something to offer. In such an environment, activities such as making sounds, singing, telling stories, or simply touching one another are especially important. In one group at the Sound View Specialized Care Center, a woman who is paralyzed on one side said, "We get together to be together. Then we do as much as we can do. It's okay."

A critical factor in creating an accepting atmosphere is the language that the therapist uses in guiding the group. For example, if the therapist were to say, "Everyone lift your right arm; now your left arm; now both arms," there might be several people who could not successfully do at least one of those activities. A person who feels obliged to do everything, in order to participate in the group, will probably drop out or otherwise resist. If directions are offered as *suggestions*, in a nonauthoritarian style, it is less likely that people will feel excluded. For example, the therapist might say, ''Can we lift one arm? How about the other arm? If you can only lift one arm, that's okay. Can anyone lift both arms? If not, lift one arm as high as you can. If you can't lift your arms, how about your fingers?'' This approach makes it possible for participants to say, ''No, I can't do this, but I can do. . .'' As group norms develop, the patients themselves might come up with suggestions for including someone with a specific physical limitation.

Implicit in dance/movement therapy is the expectation that participants will attempt to move—an expectation that stimulates patients' feelings about their bodies and their physical limitations. The authors have observed that sometimes patients feel stupid or humiliated when they cannot do a movement ''well.'' By creating a safe environment and not avoiding patients' difficulties, the therapist learns to tolerate patients' feelings about their disabilities, thus establishing a model for the group; people subsequently begin to talk about their limitations and be more supportive toward one another.

Emotionally Disturbed. More and more nursing homes are receiving patients diagnosed as psychologically disturbed. This is due partially to deinstitutionalization trends, which are emptying large state mental hospitals, and partially to physicians and families who are becoming increasingly aware of emotional disturbances in older people. Significant differences exist between the elderly person who is clinically depressed because of the sudden onset of a traumatic illness or the loss of a spouse and the older person with a long history of psychiatric disturbance. In the former case, the dance/movement therapy group can provide an opportunity for the patient to mobilize feelings of anger and frustration, express them through acceptable group activities, and gain support and validation through the sharing of these feelings. In the latter case, a person with chronic psychological problems can benefit from a dance/ movement therapy program that offers a consistent, orienting environment within a social atmosphere.

Patients with longstanding emotional disturbances are often receiving antipsychotic or antidepressant medications. Proper medication management—combined with a structured interpersonal environment—often helps such patients maintain adaptive functioning and prevents further social withdrawal and regression. Dance/movement therapy has traditionally proven to be effective treatment for long-term psychiatric patients because of the opportunities it affords for unison rhythmic movement, channeled expressions of emotions, and socialization (Chaiklin & Schmais, 1979; Samuels, 1973).

Mentally Alert. Many residents of nursing homes are mentally alert but require nursing care for physical illnesses or injuries. Some do not require total care but live in an intermediate care facility or a skilled nursing facility because they are unable to find other suitable living arrangements. Often the traditional passive entertainment and recreational activities do not adequately stimulate the mentally alert person struggling to maintain functioning. Dance/movement therapy sessions that activate the body and mind through creative and expressive involvement can provide the necessary stimulation. Approaches that encourage patient autonomy and leadership are especially appropriate for such people (e.g., helping one another get to the group, taking turns leading exercises, choosing a name for the group, and involvement in group decision-making).

After patients learn a repertoire of movements, they can exert more leadership in the group's activities. The therapist, by assuming a non-directive but warm stance, becomes a resource person for the group rather than the sole authority. The therapist may suggest new movements or creative activities but should be responsive to patient's offerings, both verbal and nonverbal. In dance/movement therapy sessions with very alert people, movement images often stimulate lengthy discussions about the past and/or present. There may be just as much talking as there is moving in such groups; this is to be expected (and even encouraged).

Contraindications

Although most people confined to a convalescent home could derive mental and physical benefits from dance/movement therapy, not all are willing or able to participate in a group experience. Some patients who are not clinically depressed and who have many visitors and adequate family support build a life for themselves in the institution within their own rooms. They are reluctant to attend most recreational or therapeutic activities yet do not appear withdrawn or isolated. Staff generally hesitate to interfere with their routine because they appear content and do not present a management problem. Such patients could benefit from an individualized exercise program to prevent muscle atrophy and maintain mobility.

Another class of patients who may not be able to benefit from group dance/movement therapy are those with paranoia. Such patients usually exhibit suspicious and guarded behavior and require very structured environments. They may be upset by imagery or expressions of emotion and may become more paranoid in a group. Sometimes very elderly people use guarded behavior as a defense against fears about their declining mental and/or physical health; attempts to disrupt their routine or involve them in new activities may be disorienting. Such patients might be able to benefit from individually administered exercise programs if the reasons for treatment were clearly communicated.

Motivation

Programs that focus exclusively on physical exercise tend to fail when presented to convalescent home patients if the exercise has no meaning for the patients and thus offers little to motivate them to activity. Many people in this situation have no motivation to improve their range of motion, stamina, breathing, or flexibility. Comments such as "We're too old to do this" or "I've exercised enough in my lifetime" are common. A rationale for activity based solely on its physiological benefits is quickly rejected by those who no longer believe that their physical health will improve.

A strong group identity—with an emphasis on addressing interpersonal needs—is a motivating factor for attending dance/movement therapy sessions. The notion that "we are a group" is a powerful force in helping people get to the sessions even when they are not feeling particularly well. Once patients enter the room, see each other, perhaps hear music, it is difficult to resist involvement.

Motivation is an issue not only for patients but also for the therapist who works in long-term care facilities. It is one thing to work at a senior center or adult education program with 50-or 60-year-olds who might prolong their independence through movement and creative expression therapy. It is quite another experience to sit in a room with 75- to 100-year-olds who can't see, hear, or speak intelligibly. In order not to be overwhelmed by feelings of pessimism and despair, it is essential in such a situation for the therapist to abandon traditional notions of cure. With rare exceptions, people are not going to get better. Often the therapist's role is not to promote cure by usual standards but to facilitate a supportive, humanizing environment in which people can express and share their fears, pleasures, and memories. Dance/movement therapy cannot cure paralysis or blindness, but it can provide a bridge for the isolation that people experience as a result of such limitations.

Establishing a Program

Until recently, there has been little demand for dance/movement therapy programs in convalescent homes. In both private and non-profit facilities, priority has been given to providing basic medical services. The combination of (1) public consciousness-raising regarding institutional care of the elderly, (2) recent legislation concerning quality of treatment in long-term care facilities, and (3) increasing interest in the relationship between activity and health has evoked great interest in movement therapy for the elderly.

Administrative Support. Adequate administrative support is essential for the success of any new program. Administrative support can be clearly demonstrated by the hiring of qualified personnel at appropriate salaries, the acquisition of adequate supplies, and the allocation of suitable space. This will concretely demonstrate to staff, patients, and families, perhaps more effectively than any rhetoric, the administration's support of the dance/movement therapy program.

The administrator should differentiate the dance/movement therapy program from other recreational and leisure activities. Although these other activities are very important in the lives of many institutionalized patients, attendance is voluntary and may be sporadic. Dance/movement therapy sessions can be viewed as part of the patient's treatment and should be presented accordingly. The staff's attitude toward the sessions influences the patients' own attitudes; if the staff considers the sessions valuable, patients are more likely to attend.

Nursing Involvement. Nursing staff cooperation is absolutely essential to the survival of any program in a convalescent facility. Nursing personnel are responsible for the minute-to-minute care and management of all patients. They, to a great extent, control whether or not someone is dressed and ready to participate in therapeutic programs. Therefore, the therapist should encourage nursing staff involvement in the dance/movement therapy sessions. Ideally, all participating staff should attend sessions regularly; however, changes in the nursing staffs' schedules are common and often make regular attendance difficult. Whenever possible, a nurse or nurse's aide should attend sessions and be encouraged to pass on any observations to other nursing staff. If nursing personnel can participate regularly, they should be invited to do so.

The dance/movement therapist must spend time with the nursing staff, in in-service programs and informal exchanges of patient data. If occasionally a patient is not ready for a session, the therapist should find out why but be sympathetic to nursing personnel's stresses. Posting a list of the dance/movement therapy groups at each nurse's station, including the day, time, place, and participants facilitates cooperation.

Personnel. Dance/movement therapy sessions should be conducted by a qualified therapist. Ideally, an assistant should participate regularly in each group, especially in groups with confused or physically disabled people. In addition to providing logistical support (transporting patients, setting up the room, etc.), a co-leader or assistant can facilitate contact with patients who have difficulty participating. Any motivated staff members or students can assist in these groups if they (1) are able to attend regularly; (2) are receptive to supervision and guidance from the dance therapist; and (3) feel comfortable moving and enjoy spontaneous interaction with patients.

At the Sound View Specialized Care Center, for example, the therapeutic recreation director, physical therapists, social workers, and college students have, at various times, assisted in the dance/movement therapy groups. In-service training and staff meetings after each session clarify the assistants' role and provide an opportunity for teaching new skills.

Size of Groups. The potential for therapeutic benefit is maximized in groups of 8 to 12 people. Certainly, creative movement activities can be beneficial to patients in large group settings; small groups, however, are more conducive to reminiscing, self-disclosure, and sharing. A comprehensive group program in a convalescent home should offer both small and large group experiences as they provide very different social environments.

Referral Criteria. Referral criteria based on cognitive functioning seem to be more important that those based on physical capabilities. For example, it is possible to have ambulatory and nonambulatory patients in the same dance/movement therapy group, but very alert people are often intolerant of confused people. In a group of less mentally alert patients, it is helpful to have people at varying levels of confusion and responsiveness. If a group comprises only extremely withdrawn, non-verbal, or nonresponsive members, the therapist will work hard, see no results, and eventually feel quite frustrated. If, however, a few people—who, despite moderate confusion—can respond to music or touch, their energy will help others become involved. In a sense, patients act as catalysts or co-therapists by creating multiple lines of communication with other patients.

Space. A private, uncluttered room that can accomodate 12 to 15 chairs and/ or wheelchairs is preferable for dance/movement therapy sessions. Recreational movement activities are often held in open lounges, but small groups are best conducted in a more protected space. This creates a safe atmosphere in which people feel free to express themselves.

CONCLUSION

An interactional approach to dance/movement therapy with the elderly can facilitate emotional expression, spontaneity, and peer interaction as well as increased bodily awareness and range of movement. Socialization is a primary goal of group approaches with convalescent home patients, along with the expression of feelings and the development of independent behavior. The isolation so prevalent in institutional settings can be alleviated by participation in group rhythmic movement activities, which lead to the sharing of feelings and memories.

Therapy facilitates recall of feelings and memories through involvement at the body level. When practiced within a setting in which group interaction and cohesion are fostered, it can provide an arena for very elderly people to express themselves and engage in social relationships. In addition to the obvious physical advantages of a regular program of activity, the psychosocial approach to dance/movement therapy offers a wide range of emotional and social benefits.

Chapter Four
Developing a Movement Therapy Program for Geriatric Patients

Susan L. Sandel

Dance or movement therapy is by no means a new modality in the treatment of geriatric patients. In 1942 Marian Chace, the founder of group dance therapy with hospitalized psychiatric patients, began working with elderly populations at St. Elizabeth's Hospital in Washington, D.C. Her students in turn carried portable phonographs into the back wards of other state mental institutions in an attempt to reach the elderly who were labeled chronically ill and for whom, in many instances, they were providing the only "treatment."

Eva Desca Garnet developed an approach to geriatric calisthenics, which became part of the physical education curriculum at the University of Southern California in 1972 (Garnet, 1972). The current national interest in the development of programs for elderly clients in convalescent homes and senior citizens' centers gives dance and movement therapists an opportunity to use skills that have been part of their training for 30 years but that they may not be applying in geriatric settings.

Increasing awareness of the psychosocial needs of elderly residents stimulated the introduction of a movement therapy program at the Sound View Specialized Care Center in West Haven in August 1976. Sound View is a 100-bed facility that maintains a reputation for high-quality individualized care. A full treatment program of physical and occupational therapy, speech therapy, and expert nursing is supplemented by extensive activities such as music, crafts, religious programs, parties, games, and other entertainment.

Originally published as "Movement Therapy With Geriatric Patients In A Convalescent Home," *Hospital & Community Psychiatry* (1978), Vol. 29, No. 11, 738-741. Copyright, 1978, the American Psychiatric Association. Reprinted by permission.

In 1976 there was a growing awareness among the staff that an emphasis on crafts, pottery, sewing, and the like is not appropriate for patients who do not have fine motor skills. These patients become extremely frustrated in activities that emphasize the completion of a product, and they often refuse to participate in any subsequent group activities. It became increasingly obvious to the Sound View professional staff that more process-oriented group experiences were needed to engage isolated individuals who, because of their severe confusion or physical limitations, were unable to participate in traditional programs.

After nine years of working with severely disturbed adolescents and young adults at the Yale Psychiatric Institute, I was interested in developing a movement therapy program with a different population. That coincided with Sound View's interest in hiring consultants for specialized programs, and I submitted a proposal for a movement therapy program to the administrators at Sound View. The primary purpose was to promote socialization through movement experiences that stimulate interaction. The physical benefits of the exercises were viewed as secondary, although simply increasing some patients' sensory stimulation would clearly be helpful. I was interested in creating an atmosphere in which individual limitations could be tolerated and any kind of expression appreciated; the most minimal participation in the group would be recognized.

The proposal contained four criteria that I thought were necessary for successful implementation of the program. They were the availability of an enclosed lounge area, a commitment from the staff to bring patients to the sessions, a consistent group of patients whose regular attendance would be encouraged by the staff, and regular participation by at least one staff member. To meet those requirements, staff would have to have a clear idea of the goals and potential value of the program.

In a convalescent home, nursing staff support is crucial for the very existence of special programs. Not only do the nursing staff prepare patients for their daily activities but they are extremely influential in conveying values and attitudes about these activities to their patients (Chace, 1975).

PREPARING FOR THE GROUP

I spent several weeks talking to staff at all levels, both individually and in groups. That orientation period culminated in a large group meeting in which the staff participated in a movement session similar to what I anticipated conducting with patients. The session stimulated the staff to think about which patients might benefit from movement therapy. I then met with the head nurses, the physical therapist, the occupational therapist, and the program director, who composed a list of potential participants—patients who were severly depressed, disoriented, and generally difficult to engage in recreational activities.

We decided that the group should consist of long-term patients since they presumably could benefit from an ongoing group experience. We tried to select patients who were unable to function in large group activities but who were thought to have potential for responding in a smaller group in which verbal participation would not be stressed.

I next attempted to talk with all those patients and selected the ones who indicated some interest or curiosity. There was some self-selection because of people who flatly refused to join on a trial basis. A group of eight men and women was formed; they ranged in age from 77 to 91, and all had been at Sound View for at least six months.

The only suitable space for the group was the staff conference room, as it was the only area that afforded any privacy. As in many facilities designed for the elderly, public areas are generally open and visible to all passers-by. I had learned from past experiences in a psychiatric hospital that it is extremely difficult to created a sense of safety and intimacy in a group that is meeting in a "fishbowl." The staff conference room was assigned to the group for one hour a week.

From the beginning I was faced with the task of setting boundaries and dealing with issues of exclusion. Besides the patients, a large crowd gathered for the first session, including several staff members, the private duty nurses and companions of several patients, and a patient with his wife and daughter; I could barely see and hear the patients. The following week I stood at the door explaining that the session was a patient group for patients to interact with one another. Some family members who wanted to attend became indignant, but most of the nurses and companions were understanding.

I asked the program director and the physical therapy director to continue to participate regularly, as they had expressed special interest. The occupational therapist offered to attend whenever necessary. By the eighth session the group had achieved cohesion; attendance was excellent except for occasional illness, and all participants indicated some investment in the group.

In November 1976 I started a second group, which consisted of seven men and women functioning at a slightly higher level. Their ages ranged from 73 to 98; some were ambulatory and quite verbal. Again the issue of exclusion emerged; for two weeks many staff and patients appeared at the wrong time for the wrong group, and I had to clearly differentiate the boundaries between the two groups. This differentiation increased everyone's curiosity about the program. Several patients were concerned about which group they were part of, particularly one man who felt that he belonged in the new group with the more alert patients. I subsequently moved him, as well as a few other patients, until the groups were more homogeneous in mental and physical functioning.

The second group had more difficulty becoming a cohesive group than the first, as indicated by fluctuating attendance and a few dropouts and discharges. However, this group also achieved considerable stability after two months, with a core of six patients.

THE MOVEMENT THERAPY SESSIONS

All the sessions begin with everyone sitting in a circle; the majority of patients are in wheel chairs. A comfortable number for our space is eight patients and two staff members; wheel chairs create a sense of crowding because of the space they require. Music is used initially to provide a rhythmic framework, although it may not be played for the entire session.

The sessions start with simple warm-up exercises involving different parts of the body; they often suggest dramatic images that I develop into group interaction. For example, in one session people took turns pulling on a long cloth rope. I suggested they add the words "Give it to me." Several participants became engaged in vigorous struggles for the rope.

I then asked if anyone fights for things they want nowadays. One man answered, "My place on the sun porch. I don't want people around. I don't want to talk, just dream." A woman answered, "What's there to fight for? There's no point." The imagery facilitated a group discussion about whether there are still things worth fighting for in life. Several people were surprised when others expressed opinions or interests similar to their own.

Such an experience gives the elderly an opportunity to share feelings and memories; they are often discouraged from such expressions by family and friends, who find the memories painful or boring. Frequently the movements in the session relate to concrete activities that trigger memories such as baking bread, rowing a boat, or rocking a baby. When people participate in movements that remind them of former competencies or pleasures, they often appear more alert, organized, and competent. Some measure of respect begins to emerge among group members, if only fleetingly, when they share former experiences of mastery.

Touch, in the form of patting, holding hands, and massage is an extremely important part of the sessions. Most patients in a convalescent home or similar setting are the passive recipients of touching—that is, they are bathed, fed, dressed, and transported by others. In the movement sessions I emphasize mutual touching, such as reaching out to hold hands or patting someone's face while being patted.

Such exercises are designed to promote the feeling of having something to give rather than exclusively receiving from others. It is difficult to encourage such feelings in a setting that fosters dependency; however, certain basic human values can be maintained despite the practical constraints. One woman said, while taking a turn at having her shoulders gently massaged by group members, "Nobody ever did this for me." Several people acknowledged that doing something for her made them feel valued in turn.

Direct physical contact often has a dramatic organizing effect on patients who drift in and out of reality. I am constantly surprised when someone who is usually disoriented makes a lucid, relevant comment while in physical contact with another person. For example, one woman characteristically sits inert, staring blankly into space. When someone holds her hand, she appears to wake up, her vacant stare changes to a smile, and she reacts appropriately to the person who is touching her. There is almost always a brief conversation between her and the other person, who also may be a patient who rarely speaks otherwise.

Besides encouraging verbalization, another major goal of the sessions is stimulating vocalization. Whenever possible I suggest accompanying movements with sounds, which may later develop into words or sentences. This technique is particularly useful for stroke patients whose speech is affected; they may participate in making group sounds in a situation that doesn't require a "correct" word. Any sound offered by a participant is welcomed and usually develops into group interaction.

It is difficult and frustrating for people in a passive, dependent position to communicate the anger or despair they may experience. The appropriate expression of aggression is tolerated in the movement therapy sessions and is supported by the use of imagery and of soft objects that can withstand abuse. When a frail looking person punches a rubber ball, he often reveals strength that has been suppressed. A woman who often weeps uncontrollably may begin talking coherently about her frustration when she is engaged in an aggressive movement. Such actions give the nonverbal patient the opportunity to communicate feelings that he may not be able to verbalize; when such feelings are internalized, they can be acknowledged and recognized as meaningful by the group.

I always comment when anyone is absent for any reason, even though the patients may not associate names with faces from week to week. If someone is ill, I explain the nature of the illness to the group. During the 17th meeting of one of the groups, a woman noticed that a man she had argued with the previous week was absent. It was the first time that anyone had spontaneously mentioned the absence of a peer. The woman was clearly disappointed that her partner was not there to engage in battle again.

When working with people who suffer from recent memory impairment, it becomes part of the routine to reiterate where we are, what we are doing, and why. Each week I must re-explain for some patients not only that it is time for movement therapy but also what it means and what we did the previous week. Although the need to repeat becomes frustrating at times, the constant reminders seem to help patients internalize at least some aspects of the group values. For example, some patients say when they see me, "Oh, it must be Wednesday." Another patient usually starts clapping her hands as soon as she enters the conference room while still asking where she is going.

CHANGES IN BEHAVIOR

During the first six months, as patients became more familiar with me and with the group structure and less self-conscious about the movement activities, I observed that spontaneous expressions of feelings occured more frequently. Several patients expressed strong affect during the sessions. There was a noticeable increase in conversation among patients before the sessions started, as well as more interaction during the sessions. For example, it was initially quite difficult for the patients to join hands; they either were unaware of others or reluctant to make contact. Most patients now hold hands willingly and help others who, because of spatial disorientation, may be having trouble locating the people next to them.

After the first two months, the assertive behavior of patients in both groups began to increase. Periodically patients began to take the lead in movement activities. They expressed negative opinions about particular exercises rather than participating in a half-hearted, compliant manner, and they sometimes took an active role in monitoring a disruptive patient's behavior.

About a month after the first movement therapy group and the open exercise class were started, Sound View staff reported changes in patients' behavior in large group gatherings. The administrator noted an increase in socialization on the sun porch and at parties. Other staff observed that patients appeared more responsive to music, and that at several events they spontaneously held hands or stood up to dance.

The program director also reported that patients seemed more willing to do exercises or creative movement activities at other recreational events. Encouraged by these results, she increased the frequency of music and movement activities, and she also added a creative art group which emphasized the creative process rather than the finished product.

The movement therapy sessions were helpful for patients by providing a structured opportunity for contact, for the sharing of life experiences and memories, and for the appropriate expression of aggression. In addition to the value of the sessions themselves, the increase in patients' socialization stimulated staff's interest in expanding the program of creative, process-oriented group activities.

Chapter Five
The Developmental Method in Drama Therapy

David Read Johnson

The use of creative arts therapy groups with the elderly is achieving increased recognition as technical and theoretical dimensions of these modalities are being described with greater sophistication. Clinical reports of verbal group therapy indicate that socialization, life satisfaction, and insight can be improved through group therapy (Benaim, 1957; Berland & Poggi, 1979; Linden, 1956). Creative arts therapies provide unique and additional benefits in group work with the elderly. Numerous reports of art, music, dance, and drama therapy in the past decade conclude that the arts therapies provide structured group interactions that elicit coherent expressions of the person's inner life. The creative arts therapies particularly benefit patients with impaired cognition by providing interpersonal structure and communication that do not rely on verbalization (Berger & Berger, 1973; Caplow-Lindner, Harpaz & Samberg, 1979; Crossin, 1976; Fersh, 1980; Gray, 1974; Weiss, 1984). In the field of drama therapy, most contributions emphasize the description of specific activities (such as exercises, plays, theatre games) and basic leadership principles (Burger, 1980; Michaels, 1981; Thurman & Piggins, 1982; Weisberg & Wilder, 1985; Ziemba, 1985). However, there is evidence that a number of coherent technical approaches based on sophisticated theoretical frameworks are emerging (Feil, 1981; Jennings, 1973). The purpose of this chapter is to articulate such a framework, identified as the Developmental Method, for drama therapy technique with the elderly. The Developmental Method is based, in part, on previous work with the elderly and other populations which has been described elsewhere (John-

Originally published in *The Arts in Psychotherapy* (1986), Vol. 13, No. 1, 17-33. Reprinted by permission of ANKHO International, Inc.

son, 1982a, 1984). After describing the technique and its theoretical rationale, I will report in detail on a complete session in order to provide a clear picture of its application with elderly patients, particularly those in nursing homes.

THERAPEUTIC GOALS

The basic goal of this form of drama therapy is to establish meaningful interpersonal relationships among group members. The therapeutic benefits of the group follow from the achievement of this goal. The activities of the group are not designed to be *specific* treatment for depression or disorientation, as antidepressant medication or reality orientation are. Nevertheless, it is expected that disorientation, interpersonal withdrawal, low self-esteem, and depression will lessen as a result of the drama therapy group.

This emphasis on interpersonal relationships is particularly important since the elderly person's struggles with issues of death and dying (Kübler-Ross, 1969), personal integrity vs. despair (Erickson, 1968), and life review (Butler, 1963) often result in an unnecessary withdrawal from others, leading to increased dysphoria and disorientation. Meaningful interpersonal relationships are established through the Developmental Method by (1) maintaining a stable and well-bounded social environment, (2) encouraging active engagement among group members through the verbal, physical, and dramatic activities, (3) utilizing reminiscence and reenactment to integrate past and present selves, and (4) openly addressing group members' physical limitations and approaching deaths. These elements are described in more detail in Chapter Two.

Other possible goals of a group therapy experience, such as providing a daily structure, developing or maintaining specific skills, gaining insight into one's personality, or effecting change in one's external environment, are not primary goals of this technique. The Developmental Method is particularly effective, however, in improving relationships by ameliorating personal fears of being incompetent, stupid or awkward, feelings of humiliation and emptiness, and the projection of these feelings through antagonistic attitudes to others ("I'm not like those ugly old people"). The result is a greater tolerance of oneself and of others, and relief from the anxieties generated by rigid interpersonal stances.

THE GROUP WITHIN THE LARGER SETTING

The institution is the context within which the elderly resident and the therapy group are embedded. For this reason, it is important that attention be given to the institution's history, current structure, and primary goals. How will the group therapy experience complement or conflict with the overall social enterprise of the nursing home? Will it be seen as a part of the regular activities program, as a special and valued activity, or as a clandestine operation? Are its goals openly supported by the authorities of management and nursing, or is it necessary for the therapist to describe the group under a different guise?

The Developmental Method that is described here is best implemented when the group therapy and therapist are seen as integrated into the nursing home community. In order for significant interpersonal relationships to be established, the residents' feelings about the nursing home must be addressed. Their identity as patient-in-the-nursing-home needs to be integrated with other identities, and this is impossible when the group or therapist represents anti-nursing home values. Development proceeds best when there is coherence and integration within the larger care-taking structure, whether that of the parents for the child, or that of therapists and staff for the elderly patient. Thus, the Developmental Method of drama therapy is enhanced by the leader's collaboration and familiarity with the nursing home.

First a period of *staff training and inservice* is required to familiarize the staff with the goals and techniques of the drama therapy group. This is followed by a *needs assessment* in which nursing and activities staff are questioned about which patients can benefit from the group, which patients are underserved, and what needs patients have that the group can address.

To establish a stable and well-bounded environment for the group, a regular time and place to meet weekly are required. The place should be a room that is a private space and is free from intrusion. A feeling of membership is reinforced by entry and departure ceremonies, and by having no unexpected visitors. Thus, patients, whether referred by staff or on their own, should be evaluated before they join the group.

Patients are best served when all function at a similar level of mental alertness and orientation, yet are heterogeneous in age, sex,

physical disability, and background. If the range in cognitive functioning is too great, the group will have difficulty establishing a
sense of cohesion. Due to the focus on interpersonal relationships,
patients are also best served if there are two therapists who can play
out different aspects of a relationship with group members and
whose relationship with *each other* can become a useful focus for
the group.

For purposes of identity and cohesion, it is helpful that the group
have a name. The name can be determined by the institution, the
therapist, or the group. Whether or not the name includes the word
"therapy" depends upon the group's relationship to the institution
and the preference of the therapist. Whatever the name, the patients
soon catch on to the therapeutic nature of the group. I do not hesitate
to use the name "drama therapy group" since it fosters an openness
about the group among the patients and staff. When the group is supported by and integrated into the larger nursing home environment
there is rarely a problem with patients avoiding the group because it
is called "therapy."

THEORETICAL BACKGROUND

The theoretical framework for the Developmental Method in drama therapy rests on two bodies of knowledge: the concept of developmental level described in theories of cognitive development
(Piaget, 1951; Werner, 1948; Werner and Kaplan, 1964) and the
concept of internalized relationships from pschoanalytic object relations theory (Guntrip, 1961; Kernberg, 1976; Klein, 1975). The
Developmental Method is applicable to drama therapy with any population since it is based on structural aspects of representation and
thought. Nevertheless, modifications of technique are required for
specific populations due to important differences in life-stage development (e.g., psychosexual, social, and moral development).

Developmental Level. Studies of cognitive development clearly
show that the developing individual matures through stages within
several dimensions of experience. The medium of representation
begins with pure sounds and movements, shifts to symbolic gesture,
then to imagery, and finally to the word (Werner & Kaplan, 1964).
The person initially relies on task, space, and role structures maintained externally by the mother or both parents, but increasingly
moves toward a state of self-reliance as s/he is capable of reproduc-

ing these structures internally (Kernberg, 1976). The ability to identify and tolerate greater complexity in one's experience increases throughout development, as does the ability to handle greater interpersonal demands from others. Finally, the capacity for containing and expressing intense affect without undue anxiety increases.

These principles of cognitive development, applied to drama therapy groups, suggest that the session be structured in a way in which ideas, images, and thoughts emerge from the group members in a developmental progression. Thus, the session should begin with sounds and movements, then utilize gesture and images, and later include role-play and verbalization; it should begin in a more structured manner and move toward less structure in its tasks, leadership, and spatial configurations; and the activities should increase in complexity, intensity of affect, and interpersonal demand. (See Johnson, 1982a, for a more detailed discussion of these concepts.)

Object Relations Theory. This theory holds that each person builds a representation of the self and others by internalizing sets of interpersonal relations (object relations) from infancy through adulthood. Initially, these relations are characterized by a lack of differentiation and integration, so that the distinction between self and other, or inside and outside, is poorly defined. As one matures, these "images" of relationships become more differentiated and accurate, and are increasingly integrated into a coherent self-image, and coherent representations of other people and the world (Kernberg, 1976). Thus, the internal world of the person consists of layers of self and other representations, some quite primitive that are derived from early experience, and others more sophisticated in form which are organized at later stages. Under stress or special environmental conditions, each person has access to these earlier forms of self/other relations. These earlier forms also tend to emerge when the media expression are of an earlier developmental level, such as sound, movement, or gesture. In fact, Schimek (1975) has suggested that the unconcious is really these early object relations contained in nonverbal forms of representation, which explains why the arts therapies are so powerful in their ability to elicit surprising and otherwise hidden parts of ourselves.

The therapist attempts to encourage the expression of representations of the self and of others. The therapist assesses whether they represent early or late versions of the self, or hopes about future selves, and to which significant others in the person's life they are attached. The medium of drama is particularly effective in evoking these representations (Johnson, 1981b). The complex internal world of each person, consisting of layers of interpersonal relations, emerges in his/her interactions with group members and the therapist, both in normal conversation and in the improvisational role-playing.

In the drama therapy group there are three worlds: the *here and now world* of the group of elderly residents and the therapists, including their actual behavior, personal characteristics, and relations with each other; the *internal world* of each participant, filled with many forms of relations between self and others; and the *external world* of family, nursing staff, and other patients to whom the group members must relate before and after the group experience. To a certain extent, the purpose of the Developmental Method is to stimulate a comingling of these worlds, so that the group serves as a safe crossroads or transitional space (Winnicott, 1971) where the internal world filled with past objects can come in contact with the external world and achieve a degree of interaction and integration. This is accomplished by introducing a new and temporary world of improvisational role-playing whose people, places, and activities become invested with aspects of the patients' real lives without being real. As a result, the role-playing serves as the vehicle for this integration of the internal and external, which is so often missing in the patient's experience in the nursing home. The fears and frustrations attendant upon entrance to the nursing home may tempt the elderly person to separate his/her .past self, filled with youthful dreams and adult accomplishments, from the anticipated hopelessness of the future self. The result is an emptying of meaning from his/her current life in the nursing home. This separation attempts to protect the self from losing the valued past. "I am *not* this crippled patient who sits here now. I am who I *was*." The drama therapy group, by utilizing techniques that evoke expressions of both the internal and the external worlds in a safe group environment where real relationships are encouraged, serves to heighten the patient's continued adaptation to and dialogue with life.

TECHNICAL CONSIDERATIONS

A number of basic principles define the therapist's technique.
Active Participation. Since the goal of the therapy is to reestablish interpersonal relationships by overcoming symptoms of depression,

withdrawal, and disorientation, the active participation of the therapist is crucial. The therapist becomes the patients' first and strongest link to other people, enticing them into engagement by playing roles that evoke memories of past attachments. S/he serves as a knowledgeable guide for the group through the mysteries and potential dangers of the dramatic medium. The therapist's activity is thus both an organizing and evocative influence in the group's environment.

Sustaining Flow. Central to the Developmental Method is the concept of flow or continuous transformation of feelings, thoughts, and group structures. Technically, each group structure should help to express the emerging inner state of the group, which is constantly changing just as the stream of consciousness of a person does. Since the nature of this ongoing transformation is spontaneous, group structures and exercises cannot be predetermined no matter how well the therapist is capable of designing an integrated sequence. Instead, in the Developmental Method, the group activity is in a constant state of transition, shifting somewhat ambiguously from one structure to another according to the therapist's understanding of the emerging imagery and movement of group members. Disruptions in this flow indicate areas of anxiety or conflict among or within group members and therapist.

The transition from one structure to another, and from one developmental level to another, entails a corresponding reorganization of the group members' relationships with each other, and each individual's connection to the group as a whole. This requires flexibility. Typically, some individuals experience anxiety during each transformation and resist it, thereby communicating important information to the therapist. By creating and maintaining an environment of constant transition and transformation, the therapist helps the group members to overcome their anxieties when faced with the necessity of change. This leads to an increase in the range and flexibility of their self-image.

The Developmental Method does not assume that a one-way movement up the developmental ladder (toward verbalization, for example) is the goal. Rather, it aims to develop the full range of expression across all modes of expression, all levels of self-representation, and to develop the ability to shift flexibly among them (Johnson, 1982a.) The therapist contributes to this effort by monitoring and sustaining the flow of the session.

Generating Hypotheses. As images, thoughts and feelings emerge during each stage of the session, the therapist needs to be alert to the potential meanings of these images for the group: meanings that may not be fully developed or conscious, and that if fully acknowledged might please or distress them. At each stage in the group process the therapist attempts to construct an idea of what is going on, continuously revising his/her understanding as the session develops. In the Developmental Method, the therapist uses this understanding to organize scenes, structure roles, and make comments that help the group to focus on its central theme. To the extent that the therapist's leadership is determined by his/her understanding of meanings rather than characteristics of the exercises, the session is more apt to follow a developmental progression that elicits the self-expression of group members. Despite its necessary inexactness, the therapist's currently-held hypothesis serves as a rudder which can keep the group on course toward the expression of important meanings. Without it, the therapist can miss the group's defenses against or detours around such expression at key moments in the session. The group may then be unable to achieve a sense of coherence or integration around the emerging issues.

Reverse Transference. The therapist needs to be aware of the complex nature of the transference in work with the elderly. The therapist is seen both as a parental figure, who is responsible for the organization, leadership, and safety of the group, and as the child, due to his/her younger age. This reverse transference (Meerloo, 1955) adds great complexity to the relationships between therapist and group in a developmentally based therapy since at any given moment either the therapist or a patient may represent the stage of higher development. Knowledge of this relationship may help the therapist decide whether to enter the role-playing as the group member's child or parent.

STAGES IN THE TECHNIQUE

The Greeting. The initial phase of the group includes gathering the patients, casual conversation, sharing of important events in their lives since last week, and reviewing what occurred last week in the group. The therapist is attentive to the themes and issues that are alluded to during this time.

The First Stage: Unison Activity. At some point in the conversation it will feel "right" to begin the opening movement ritual. Often a patient will initiate it. **Sound and Movement** is an opening ritual in which each member leads the group in a simple exercise or movement with an accompanying sound, such as raising a hand and saying "Ahhhh!" The group keeps the action going as each member in turn leads the group with their own sound and movement. **Vowels** is another ritual in which the group sings out each vowel (a, e, i, o, or u) several times in unison with accompanying movements. In **Impulses**, the group holds hands and passes a squeeze around the circle and then adds sounds.

The sounds and movements are repeated many times as alterations and intonations are introduced. Thus, the simple raising of an arm becomes more of a reach *for* something. The "Ahhhh" becomes more of an "Ahhhh, ha!" The singing of "uuuuuuu" sounds more like "you!" That is, each sound and movement becomes imbued with nascent imagery of feelings and objects. Pure sound approaches early forms of speech, the movements become gestures, and the empty air becomes filled with mimed "things."

At this point there is typically some anxiety because what is emerging from the group is somewhat primitive, yet ambiguous and unformed. There is pressure to define it. Defined at the correct time, it will express and contain significant parts of the members' internal lives; defined prematurely, it will serve to avoid awareness of these meanings. The correct timing is always made clear by the burst of energy and often surprise that the group experiences when an apparently random action takes on an unexpected, but familiar, meaning.

Stage Two: Defining. As each member takes turns leading the group's unison activity and offers imagery, the therapist can quickly identify by the response of the group which developing image seems to express a group theme. This is helpful to the therapist in constructing an hypothesis about the salient concerns or conflicts that the group is attempting to express that day. At this point the therapist can make three kinds of suggestions that help in defining these issues further. **Pairing**: Here the therapist says, "Now direct that to your neighbor," and each person turns to his/her neighbor and directs the sound and movement there. This usually evokes more specific imagery and intonation concerning others, leading to further transformation. **Going Around**: The therapist says, "Pass that sound and movement around the circle," and, one at a time, each person performs the action, often giving it new meanings. As the action moves around the circle, the therapist can choose to develop any particular intonation or meaning in which the group indicates an interest. **Identifying**: The therapist can also say: "What or who does this remind you of? What could this be?" Various group members will offer different ideas, each of which can be picked up on and used to transform the action further. Each of these techniques can be used many times as the group moves toward the expression of a particular set of feelings and roles that concern them that day. The therapist facilitates the transformation both by picking up on the most salient group theme, and by developing hypotheses about what the underlying theme or issue is, and how each group member might experience it differently. Going Around allows each group member to offer specific variations on the theme. Pairing evokes the different interpersonal meanings of the action. Identifying increases the articulation or fullness of the image.

The actions and images are in this way continuously transformed, moving around and around the group, and from one movement to another. For a while a particular image may be developed, or one person may keep the focus, but then variations are introduced and the therapist will facilitate the transition to these new underlying images initiated by other group members. As the group's images become increasingly defined, a pattern emerges more and more clearly, with vague feelings and objects turning into specific feelings between two or more people. For example, the "Ahh, ha" is added to a finger pointing action, and slowly the figures of a scolding parent and naughty child caught with his hand in the cookie jar may emerge.

Personification. The next stage involves the temporary crystallization of these images into differentiated roles, or characters, linked by an affective bond in an emerging "scene." The richness of these pre-character representations is impressive due to the fact that they are derived from multiple sources. These images may refer to people from the patients' past lives, alive in their reminiscences; they may also refer to aspects of their relationships to the therapist and other group members. Finally, they may also refer to people in their lives in the nursing home or family, the people of their external world. These three worlds, internal, the here and now, and external, are co-present sources of the emerging scenes. Thus, the scolding parent and naughty child image may represent memories of themselves as children or memories of themselves as parents, or feelings about the strict therapist, or about themselves as older parents of the young and untrustworthy therapist, or of their fears of the nursing staff, or their desire to scold a careless aide.

Any one of these contexts can become the content of the ensuing role-play. This transition from the ambiguous and fleeting images of the early part of the session to the more overt and structured role-play is a crucial point in the session. What guides the decision by the therapist is not what the group's image "really" means, since an image has meaning at all of these levels, but the clinical intuition and hypotheses of the therapist in determining which context is currently the most salient and the one that the group will derive the most benefit from exploring. This period therefore deserves to be given a significant amount of time, though it is often tempting for the therapist to move too quickly from a developing image in the unison activity phase to a structured role-play. Unfortunately, this bypasses an important transitional phase in which the various fragmented meanings offered by group members are transformed into a collective group image of greater power.

A technique that provides a flexible structure for this phase is called the **Magic Box**. After the group has established several images and is on the verge of moving into structured role-play, the therapist or a group member may request that the Magic Box be brought down. The Magic Box is an imaginary box, usually stored in the ceiling, which contains anything that the group wishes as well as the contents of all previous sessions. The Box is always treated with great reverence. The group members bring it down by raising their arms slowly toward the ceiling and giving a loud hum in unison as they lower their arms. Then the lid is slowly unscrewed by the group, with accompanying groans of exertion. Following this, the group is encouraged to look over the edge of the Box and to peer into it. The therapist can leave the contents of the Box unstructured, simply saying, "What do people see? What's in there?" More often the therapist, based on his/her hypothesis about the current group issues, suggests that group members each take something out of the Box. What is taken out is often a feeling, an object, a wish, a person, a sound, a movement, a mask, or a memory. These are shown and described by each member to all the others. They can then be passed around, given to a partner, or articulated further; that is, the therapist can apply the same techniques for defining as above, noticing which images evoke the greatest interest and energy from the group as a whole.

Two techniques are useful in maintaining the flow of images produced by the Magic Box. One is to have group members return their
images to the Magic Box and then repeat the process. For example,
the Box may become an **Emotional Soup**. Group members take
turns removing an emotion from the Box and leading the whole
group in showing it (e.g., by growling and grimacing for "Anger").
Then the group puts that emotion back in the soup and someone else
pulls out another one. The other technique is called the **Zap**. Group
members place all of the images that they have taken from the Box
into the center of the group and, with their hands and feet, stir them
together. The group often describes this as a "mess." The therapist
tells them that the group has tremendous power to transform this
"mess" into something completely different by working together
and "Zapping" it. The group then lowers their arms and begins a
"zzzzzing" sound which increases in volume as their arms are raised
above their heads, leading to a loud "ZZaappp!!" as they throw
their arms quickly out toward the center of the group. In the hush
that usually follows, the therapist may ask what people see, or
"what has it turned into now?" The group can then again take objects, feelings, etc., from the center.

Occasionally the group finds it difficult to personify their images.
A particularly powerful technique that can aid in transforming
divergent feelings and images into a representation of a person is
called **Creating a Person**. The therapist begins by noticing with
great interest that a person is in the·Magic Box. The therapist indicates that the person is familiar to all the group members, and,
picking this person out of the Box, s/he says "Hi!" and engages in a
short conversation with him/her. The person is referred to as
"you," "my son," or "Mom," etc., but with little articulation.
This person is passed around the group, and each member in their
conversation is asked to describe one additional attribute of the person, such as name, age, family, work, feelings, problems, or
wishes. The person is passed around until s/he is fully articulated.
Then the therapist builds a structured role-play around the character
and his/her life. The person, as the group's creation, often represents important aspects of members' lives.

These dramatic structures allow the group to develop and
transform a variety of images that express themes with interpersonal
dimensions. The feeling of anger becomes anger at *someone*, the
memory is about *someone*, the object becomes the gift from *someone*. When the basic pattern of roles has emerged in the session the

therapist can lead the group into a focused role-play involving these roles. Usually these roles are explored in a structured format, provided by the therapist, in which group members play different characters in a scene. Later the role-playing will move to more unstructured formats.

Structured Role-Playing. This phase emerges smoothly from the previous stage and is a time for greater focus on one set of object relations that are of concern for the group members. Depending upon how the therapist has facilitated the personification of the group's imaging, the roles will either remain at a "made-up" level, or will be people from patients' memories (such as parents), or from their current living situation. Various scenes may be played, with different patients taking part, often taking turns at the two or three basic roles. Discussion and reminiscing are interspersed with the scenes, which are articulated in personal ways for each participant. The therapist may play a role with each person in turn, or each person may talk to an empty chair placed in the middle of the group, or a group drama may be constructed. In **Phoning Home**, for example, a group member "calls" a significant other in his/her family. The therapist plays the operator who connects the person to the people in his/her life, played by other group members.

The therapist is often tempted in this stage to focus exclusively on one issue or one person, as in psychodrama, or to turn the role-plays into a form of problem-solving. In the Developmental Method these are not goals of the session. The purpose of this structured phase is to intensify the group's central theme so that past and current conflicts and anxieties are explored within the group process. This is expected to lead to a smooth transition into the next phase where the therapist helps the group move to a more complex and less structured format characterized by flexibility and transformation, that is, play. If the structured role-play becomes too concentrated on one person this transition is interfered with, since what was originally the group's issue has been placed in an individual.

Unstructured Formats: Playing. In the previous phase, images were crystallized in the form of structured roles and scenes. Now the group's images are allowed greater room again, though often the focus on past figures shifts to the patients' current relationship to the therapist and other group members. This is accomplished through three techniques.

1. **The Therapist as Subject**. The therapist enters into the role-play by picking up on a comment of a group member and transform-

ing it into a new scene. The therapist purposely takes on a role that is consistent with the transferential image of him by group members (e.g., the strong parent figure, the naughty child), and then casts the patient in the complementary role (consistent with the original comment). If the therapist's empathy is accurate, there is usually a burst of energy or laughter. The similarity of the role-play with the members' actual feelings about the therapist often leads to a playful awareness on their part about these feelings. The therapist now establishes him/herself as the focal point of the playing, often by being the one who is the cause of the problem, and thereby anchors the spontaneity that is to follow.

2. **Expanding the Scene**. The therapist might play the son while a group member plays his father. As this scene proceeds, the therapist simply turns to another group member (up to this point an audience member) and addresses him/her as another character, such as his mother ("Mother, tell Dad that I didn't do that"). Group members quickly learn to respond to this invitation and, if role and person are appropriately matched, they enter the role-play with great energy. In this way, other group members are brought in, as brothers, neighbors, teachers, uncles, etc., creating a mini-society. Once the group members learn this structure, they too begin to spontaneously cast each other in roles. As the scene continues to transform, the "problem" person may change as conflicts among other characters become more interesting or relevant to the group. This is a simplified version of the technique of **Transformation** which is used with other populations (Johnson, 1984). The scene usually moves to a pitch of energy and spontaneity before members begin to tire. At this point, the therapist may allow the group to move toward closure or may initiate the following technique.

3. **Psycho-opera** (Klein, 1979). The therapist simply begins to sing his words, usually in an exaggerated manner similar to opera, signalling others in the play to do so as well. Choral responses, sounds of the orchestra, and gesturing accompany the ensuing interaction, which often departs from the previous scene. The spontaneity of the exercise usually incites group members into saying how they feel about one another, the session, and the therapist. It is rare for this opera to last long, and, as people tire, the therapist can lead them into a choral humming or group mime of an orchestra concluding the piece.

Closing Ritual. As the group finishes its playing or opera, characterized by rather direct expressions of how they feel about each other, they often burst into applause, becoming for a moment the audience that has viewed their performance. The need to close the group in a structured and safe manner requires a verbal discussion and checking in with each member as well as a unifying closing ritual that signals the end of the session. Often, when the Magic Box has been used, all of the material produced by the group is put back into it and its lid is screwed on. Then the group moves it back into the ceiling with arm motions and a hum, waving goodbye until the next session. The discussion allows each group member to raise concerns, questions, or make comments on the session and what it meant to him or her. Finally, the therapist may remind the group about any announcements made at the beginning of the group. Then the group members take hands and, as they raise them, they all shout the name of the group in unison.

I will now present an actual session which illustrates the Developmental Method described here. The group consists of six nursing home residents, aged 80-94, who are oriented with moderate cognitive impairments. All are confined to wheelchairs due to limb amputation, arthritis, or stroke. One has had a diagnosis of schizophrenia. Two are nearly deaf. All are in stable condition. The group has met weekly for two years.

A DRAMA THERAPY SESSION

Greetings

TH: How are people feeling today?
ANNA: Lonely. I'm very lonely.
AGNES: Now? In the drama group?
ANNA: Not now.
TH: What is different about the group, Anna?
ANNA: I know the people here.
JOHN: You mean all of us good looking men! (laughter)
LILLIAN: At least you are congenial.
CHARLIE: I should hope so.
TH: How about other people?
ROSE: I'm thinking about the holiday.
    (Group discussion about the upcoming holiday, including what they will be served for dinner. There is no mention of their children or relatives visiting.)

Unison Activity

TH: Why don't we start. Who'd like to lead off? [SOUND/MOVE-MENT]

JOHN: (Begins a double arm movement outward, which the group joins.) Whee! . . . Whee! (joyous tone) . . . Whee (more declaratory) . . . We! (as the arms move out they seem to refer to the group members) . . . We! (then as the arms return, John initiates) . . . You! (one arm pointing into the center) . . . We! . . . You! . . . We! . . . You!

TH: (On "You," he points towards a member of the group; others follow.) We! . . . You! (acquires an ominous, accusatory tone). (As the sound and motion continues) Whose turn now? (Several people point at someone and say "You," laughter.) Ok, Anna.

ANNA: Ahhh! (changes the movement to a slow opening wide of the arms)

GROUP: Ahhh! Ahhh! Ahhh!

Defining

TH: Direct it toward someone! (Group directs their arm movement toward each other.) [PAIRING]

GROUP: Ahh! (more harsh) Ahh! (movement changes to one arm striking out at each other) Ahh, *ha*! Ahh, *ha*!

ROSE: You caught me!

LILLIAN: I didn't do it!

JOHN: Is this my hand in the cookie jar?

GROUP: (Continues) Ahh, ha! (laughter)

[The therapist notices the energy that this image elicits from the group, and decides to "poll" group members for specific variations.]

TH: Let's pass that around the circle. Agnes, direct that movement and sound toward Anna. [GOING AROUND]

GROUP: (One at a time, each member directs the movement toward his/her partner. Members show childlike manners, as if they are children who have been caught by their parents.)

TH: What does this remind you of? [IDENTIFYING]

JOHN: When I was caught playing hooky from school.

GROUP: Ahh, ha!

CHARLIE: Ding, dong, school's starting.

LILLIAN: I was never late for school.

[The therapist senses that this school image holds importance for group members, and so attempts to facilitate its development into personified roles.]

Personification

TH: Who'd like to be the teacher?

CHARLIE: Come on, you'll be late, you'll have to stay after school.

ROSE: I'm coming! I was too busy playing jacks. My father would get upset. "Jacks is not the most important thing," he would say. You couldn't answer my father. He never touched us, but he would scold.

JOHN: When I misbehaved, he took out the old hickory stick.

ROSE: Maybe it worked better than scolding.

JOHN: Take us to the principal. "Hold out your hand." (He holds out his hand to Charlie, who pretends to slap it with a ruler.) Ohh!

TH: Let's all put out our hands in the center and receive our punishment for being tardy. [UNISON]

GROUP: Ohh! Ohh!

ANNA: (to Agnes) What did you do wrong?

AGNES: I was late.

ANNA: Naughty girl.

[The therapist at this point is unaware of the possible link between this scene and the patients' concerns about their own children being tardy in visiting them for the holiday. Feeling confused, he nevertheless continues to allow the conflict to develop.]

TH: Let's go around the circle and each person take a turn being caught for being late to school. [GOING AROUND]

AGNES: Charlie, you were late for school.

CHARLIE: I'm sorry, I'm sorry . . . Now it's my turn!

JOHN: (To Charlie) I didn't mean to be late.

CHARLIE: Out to the woodshed!

JOHN: Ohh! This is like being pledged to my fraternity. They said, "Assume the position" and then whacked you in the behind! (He demonstrates.)

ROSE: (To Lillian) You were naughty.

LILLIAN: I know, I couldn't help it. (To therapist) You're so bad! You're always late! Why can't you be on time?

TH: I'm sorry, it will never happen again. I promise. (Group tension increases at this point.)

[The therapist was also tense. He had been late for a few sessions, but that had been several months ago. Yet Lillian's comments communicated an anger that was sincere. Confused, he did nothing.]

CHARLIE: Ding, dong! School's out. (He pulls his arm in a downward motion as if he was ringing the bell.)

TH: Let's join Charlie in ringing the bell.

GROUP: Ding, dong! . . . Dong. . . . Dong. . . (as the arms go up, the group adds a sound) Oh! . . . Dong. . . . Oh. . . Dong . . . . Oh! (As if something wonderful is above.)

TH: What is it?

AGNES: Sky. Wonderful sky.

JOHN: A big white cloud.

GROUP: Ohh!

LILLIAN: I want that rainbow.

GROUP: Ohh!

[The therapist now perceives the clear separation between "being bad" (as the bad children) and "good" represented by the sky imagery, which is "out there." He now attempts to help the group bring the good in.]

TH: Ok, lets take all that good up there, the sky, the white cloud, and the rainbow, and whatever else there is and bring it down, all together, bring it down and into ourselves (indicates by bringing arms down onto chest. Group follows in unison.)

ANNA: (Pats herself on the chest)

TH: Yes, let's pat ourselves.

ROSE: I don't deserve it.

TH: You don't deserve to be cared for?

ROSE: Half the time they don't mean it. They give you a pat, and say, "Looking good!" and then forget it. Oh well, take it from whence it comes.

ANNA: Can be the doctor too. Sometimes he just says it. You think they mean everything they say.

GROUP: (General agreement expressed)

TH: You mean people who visit you often try to say something optimistic, but it doesn't feel real to you.

ROSE: It's not that they are lying on purpose.

CHARLIE: The doctor gets his $20.

TH: Let's go around and show us what you mean. Take turns being the doctor. [GOING AROUND]

GROUP: (Group members take turns saying, "Looking good" in a false way to each other around the circle.)

[The therapist guesses that the group's insistence on holding onto the bad is in the service of preserving the good for others on whom they depend, such as doctors, or their children. He now feels comfortable enough to structure a specific role-play on the issue.]

Structured Role-Play

TH: OK, Agnes, why don't you play the doctor, and Rose, you be the patient, only as the scene goes along, turn toward us and tell us what you really feel inside about it.

AGNES: (As Doctor) You are looking very good, Rose.

ROSE: (To group) If she only knew. But I take it from whence it comes. (To Agnes) Thank you, Doctor.

AGNES: You're welcome.

ROSE: But why does my hip hurt?

AGNES: I don't know. We're depending on time to cure. It takes time, my dear.

ROSE: Yes, doctor.

TH: So what do you really think, Rose?

ROSE: I think he's a liar. But I have to have him. Whether you want to or not, if you don't call him, they wonder what's wrong. So you call him and don't listen.

TH: You don't listen?

JOHN: Yes, but it's a secret. Don't tell.

CHARLIE: Shh.

ROSE: Shh.

TH: Shh.

GROUP: Shh! (Repeat this to each other. Many smiles.)

LILLIAN: Let's bring down the Magic Box.

TH: Yes, it sounds like it's time. OK, group, with the power which we have, let's bring down the Magic Box from the ceiling. [MAGIC BOX]

GROUP: (Slowly raise arms in unison toward ceiling and then lower them.) Hmmmmmmm. (Then group mimes unscrewing the lid.)

TH: (Looking into the Box) What's in there today?

ANNA: Secrets.

[The therapist realizes that the group has many secrets that they would like to express, though they needed to back off from the previous scene which criticized the doctor. Guessing that the important feelings are associated with their families, he takes on a parental image.]

TH: (in mock parental tone) If I ever find out what you kids have done, you'll be in big trouble! (laughter)

ROSE: Look, I see a fish here. (She forms a ''fish'' with her hands and pretends to swim.)

GROUP: (Others mimic her movements.)

ROSE: When this fish finds another smaller fish, he gobbles him up. (She grabs Anna's hands.)

ANNA: Splash!

TH: Let's all splash.

GROUP: Splash! . . . Splash! (They pretend to splash each other playfully.) Splash! Splee. . . lasshh! Lash! Lash! (Movement is changed to a lashing movement, as if a whip were being held by both hands. Nervous laughter.)

TH: You bad, bad child!

CHARLIE: I remember when my father lashed me. I was supposed to have done the chores for him, and I didn't. He was very disappointed in me.

LILLIAN: One time I was twelve and I stole a candy bar from the pantry and put it in my pocket before we went to church. It was a hot day, so it melted all over my dress. My mother was so embarrassed. I looked like a mess.

TH: Sounds like some of the secrets are coming out.

(Other group members begin to reminisce about childhood memories in which they disappointed their parents.)

JOHN: My father worked in a machine shop. Worked all day. He only had a couple of hours off. I used to feel so sad for my mother. But now I realize how happy we were. We would have a big Sunday dinner after he scolded us. We never saw him during the week, so he had to scold us on Sunday before our dinner. My mother made such a wonderful dinner, though sometimes we had to eat standing up (smiles).

TH: Charlie, why don't you be John as a child, and, John, you play your father. Show us how he scolded you.

JOHN: Son, you've been bad this week. You haven't helped your mother enough. After we're gone, you are going to have to take care of yourself. We won't live forever!

CHARLIE: I know, Dad.

JOHN: I'm always right, aren't I?

CHARLIE: Yes, Dad. (John pretends to slap Charlie's hand as punishment.) Ouch!

JOHN: That's the way it was!

TH: You really looked up to your Dad, didn't you?

JOHN: Yes, I did . . . at least until he died.

TH: How did he die?

JOHN: He worked himself to death. I was still young when he died.

TH: He never got to see how you did as an adult?

JOHN: (very sad) No, he didn't.

TH: I wonder what he would think about your life.

JOHN: I do too.

TH: Perhaps we will phone him, wherever he is, up there, and ask him? Who'd like to call John's father? [PHONE HOME]

CHARLIE: I will. (Pretending to phone) Rringg. Rringg.

[The therapist, sensing a great deal of emotion in John, offers some comic relief to lighten the atmosphere so the scene does not intimidate other members.]

TH: (In nasal tone of an operator) Yes. Who are you calling?

CHARLIE: John's Dad, in Heaven.

TH: Is this a collect call? No, OK.

JOHN: Hello, John, how are you?

CHARLIE: Fine, Dad. I wanted to ask you what you thought about my life.

JOHN: I thought you'd turn into a bum for sure, but you have done all right for yourself. I have to admit I'm surprised.

CHARLIE: I wish you had been here to see it, Dad. We never had much time together. I've worked really hard.

JOHN: That you have, my boy—though I did too, and look what happened to me!

CHARLIE: I miss you. Goodbye.

TH: Would anyone else like to call their parents?

(Other members take turns calling their dead parents. Most are matter-of-fact conversations, except for Anna, who becomes tearful in telling her mother that she misses her. A general discussion and more sharing of memories follows.)

AGNES: (To therapist) Now its your turn! You have been thinking about other things. Pay attention!

[The therapist notices that the group members have not felt comfortable to express their angry feelings towards their children or parents during the entire session, continuing to take a depressive or

victimized stance. Agnes now expresses this anger by displacing it
onto the therapist, presumably a safer target. The therapist hopes
to address this displacement by responding in a role that matches
the true object of the patients' anger— in effect, by offering an action interpretation.]

Unstructured Format

TH: (Speaking to her in a whining voice) Mom, I'm sorry I didn't
visit you last month, you know how busy I am. [TH AS SUBJECT]

AGNES: (Recognizing that the therapist has initiated a role-play)
Well, David! You have been very negligent. Why haven't you
visited?

TH: Shelly and I have been very busy. You wouldn't want me to
risk my career just to visit you?

AGNES: (Outraged) Just to visit your mother! Insolent child. You
should show greater respect for your parents!

TH: Besides (indicating John), my brother Bill visits you all the
time.

AGNES: Who?

TH: You know, Bill, your favorite son. [EXPANDING ROLE-
PLAY]

JOHN: (Accepting the role) You've always been a problem in our
family. You don't show any respect or appreciation for your
parents.

AGNES: Yes, Bill dear, you do appreciate us (smiles at John).

TH: But I appreciate you too, isn't that right, Shelly? (indicating
Rose)

ROSE: Yes, David cries every night because he loves you so.

JOHN: He sure doesn't show it!

TH: (To Charlie) Dad, I think Mom is being too harsh on me.

CHARLIE: No she isn't. We haven't seen you in weeks. Where
have you been? She's a sick woman and you don't even care.

(In the same way, Lillian is brought in as Bill's wife, and Anna
becomes David's grandmother.)

TH: (falsely) I think she's looking good.

CHARLIE: I'm very disappointed in you, son.

TH: You always liked Bill better. At least Grandma likes me, right
Grandma?

ANNA: Yes, my dear, you're a good child.

(The scene develops into a heated argument, with David receiving much criticism for his obnoxious attitude. In the end, he leaves his wife to stay with his grandmother who is the only one who can tolerate him. As the story ends, there is laughter and some applause.)

TH: That was quite a scene.

ANNA: Children today don't appreciate their parents like we did.

[Rather than helping the patients verbalize their angry feelings about their children, which he intended to do, the therapist now redirects them toward their loving feelings for their parents. The patients then temporarily resume externalizing the "good" and internalizing their bad and empty feelings.]

TH: I can tell you loved your mother and father very much.

ANNA: Yes, I do.

TH: They're gone now.

ANNA: Many years ago. A long time.

ROSE: But it feels like yesterday that they were here. It was the most painful thing to lose them. I'll never get used to it.

ANNA: My father is dead now a long time. No use talking. How long can you mourn after the dead?

TH: Lillian, you are feeling something now?

LILLIAN: (crying) I miss them. They were so good. They took care of me, watched over me. . . .

TH: You have your children.

LILLIAN: Yes, and grandchildren, but it's not the same. . . . I don't know.

CHARLIE: My parents died 35 years ago. I took care of them for a long while.

TH: Lillian, did you have to care for them at the end?

LILLIAN: Yes, but it didn't do much good.

ROSE: God takes us all when he decides. (A long tense silence)

CHARLIE: You're a strong person, Lillian.

LILLIAN: (smiling) I wouldn't have lived so long if I wasn't strong! (Laughter)

[On their own, Charlie and Lillian have pointed out that they are not completely sad, weak, and lost souls, even though they have suffered losses. Her humor, in reasserting the integration of good and bad, results in a burst of energy within the group. The therapist, back on track, now encourages more spontaneous expression by introducing psycho-opera.]

TH: (singing in a mock operatic voice) Oh, you wouldn't have lived

so long, if you weren't so strong, so strong! . . . From now on
we sing instead of talk. [PSYCHO-OPERA]

JOHN: (singing) She's a strong old ladeee!

TH: (leading the chorus) Strong old lady! Strong old lady!

LILLIAN: I've lost my mo-ther!

GROUP: Oh, no! (They now add sound effects mimicking trumpets
and drums.) Boom, boom, boom.

LILLIAN: And I've lost my father!

GROUP: Oh, no! Boom, boom, boom.

CHARLIE: And God has taken them all to a safe haven, safe haven.

GROUP: Hallelujah! Hallelujah! (Laughter) Bruagghh! Bruagghh!

ANNA: But I am lonely.

TH: Oh, we are all, so lonely.

ROSE: Our children don't visit us enough.

GROUP: Visit us, visit us! Boom, boom, brannnggg!

TH: Parents gone, children gone, I'm the only one around.

AGNES: No, you're not! You're only here once a week.

GROUP: Once a week, once a week!

LILLIAN: And he takes vacations.

GROUP: VACATIONS . . . VACATIONS!

TH: You're not being fair.

GROUP: Life isn't fair. Life isn't fair!

TH: I guess you're right, life isn't fair.

GROUP: Ha-le-lu-jah! Ha-le-lu-jah! (applause)

TH: Each person take a bow! (Each person leans forward while others clap. There is a moment of relaxed silence. John holds Lillian's
hand.)

TH: If only your children came to visit. If only your parents were
still alive. That *would* be a fair trade for the love you have for
them.

CHARLIE: Are you still lonely, Anna?

ANNA: I know you care for me, Charlie. (To therapist) Where are
you going for the holiday?

TH: Sounds like you have been wondering how much I care about
the group too? (Smiling) Actually, I'm not going anywhere this
time. We will have the group next week as always . . . But, if
you prefer . . .

JOHN: Sure, go ahead. We don't need you! (Laughter)

TH: That would be pretty embarrassing, to need someone a third
your age?

AGNES: A baby! . . . Pipsqueak!

TH: Mom! (Laughter) Well, I don't think we will be able to resolve this problem today.

Closing Ritual

TH: Let's put everything back in the Magic Box. What do we have?
ROSE: My parents.
AGNES: Sadness.
TH: Put it in (points to the Box in the center of the circle). What else?
JOHN: My lashing.
LILLIAN: My memories.
CHARLIE: My bad son, David.
TH: Yes let's all put him in. (They do so with pleasure.) Now, let's put that lid back on and, with the power of the group, let's begin a hum and lift it back into the ceiling for safe keeping. Okay? Here goes . . .
GROUP: Hmmmmm (Lift arms toward ceiling).
TH: Say goodbye.
GROUP: Goodbye (waving).
TH: What did people think about today's session?
(Group members briefly report that they enjoyed it, particularly the scene with the therapist as the bad son. Several again bring up the holiday and talk about their families visiting.)
TH: Our time is up for today.
GROUP: (The group holds hands and as they lift them up they chant) Drama Group! Drama Group! Drama Group!

This group continued for five years. The members developed very intense, positive relationships with each other which sustained a sense of play and warmth. They as well as the therapist benefited greatly from this group, through which they held firmly to an appreciation of life and learned to forgive themselves for some of their own faults.

DISCUSSION

This case example demonstrates the Developmental Method with an established group of nursing home residents who were familiar with the therapist and drama therapy. At the time of the session the group had been meeting for two years and had overcome initial resistances to role-playing, fantasy, and the spontaneous atmosphere. They had also become comfortable sharing their personal feelings with each other, though the major interpersonal exploration was focused on their relationship with the therapist.

The session's major theme centered on the patients' resentment arising out of their dependency on their children, who they feared did not love them sufficiently, and secondarily upon the therapist, to whom they looked for care. However, to express the anger directly toward these figures risked retaliation or abandonment. Over the course of the session, they were able to express this anger more directly without becoming overwhelmed with feelings of guilt or fear of abandonment. The therapist's use of humor supported a sense of safety in the session by reassuring the members that he could tolerate the increasingly intense emotion. Both the humor and the role-playing provided a buffer in which the feared emotions and interactions were tested. Group members initially preferred to absorb the bad feelings by representing themselves as weak, sick, and naughty, and to idealize the therapist and their parents. At first, the therapist did not understand these images of naughtiness and punishment presented by the group. Gradually, as the dramatic images were defined and personified, the major themes involving their family members, and himself in the transference, emerged. The deaths of their parents obviously still haunted them, indicated by the regrets and expressions of guilt that were voiced. The loss of their parents required the patients to turn to their children and the therapist to meet their dependency needs, subjecting them to feelings of embarrassment and resentment.

In the last part of the session, the therapist was uncertain whether to continue to focus on the patients' feelings of loss or to help them express their anger at the children. When Charles and Lillian indicated that they were capable of tolerating the idea that, while they had suffered, they were still strong, he was able to lead the group into a spontaneous opera that allowed for more direct expressions of aggression.

Overall, this session followed a developmental progression which I have described in a previous paper (1982a). The level of structure began at a very high level and slowly decreased to allow for more spontaneous expression and control by group members. The level of complexity of the exercises increased from unison group activities to role-plays with differentiated roles, to highly complex improvisations in which people shifted roles. The developmental level of the media moved from pure sound and movements, to images, then verbal role-plays, discussion, and finally improvisations in which pure sounds, images, and words were interspersed. The interpersonal demand of the activities increased from low levels to intense contact and interaction, and the expression of affect began at a humorous, superficial level and moved to more intense and distressing affects. The anxieties aroused in the key transition points at the beginning and end of the session were contained by group rituals, and familiar group events (like the Magic Box) were used to structure more intense parts of the session. Thus, drama therapy serves a differentiating function by simplifying and concretizing feeling states and interpersonal relationships. Group members become more able to identify and structure aspects of their experience, which increases their sense of personal control as well as their capacity to verbalize.

The Developmental Method facilitates the unfolding of the murky, ambiguous, and shifting feelings of the group into more coherent, concrete group themes and issues. The therapist is constantly developing hypotheses about the meaning of the group's activities and uses this understanding to choose structures through which the issues will emerge more clearly. From an object relations view, the session demonstrates how the improvisational role-playing becomes symbolized as a projective container of the patients' psychological worlds. The characters and relationships in the role-playing come to represent the patients' past relationships, here-and-now relationships with the group and transference to the therapist, and relationships with family and nursing staff. The safety of the group's structure encourages them to place these parts of themselves into the dramatic images and scenes which serve as transitional containers. The Magic Box is the most explicit example of this holding function of drama. The initial period of intense projection is eventually followed by periods of re-introjection during which the group members take these parts of themselves back, only in a modified form: (1) in that they have been expressed, they are now conscious; (2) in that they have been shared in a group format, they have been modified by social interaction; and (3) in that the therapist has maintained the level of anxiety at manageable levels, they are modified in intensity. The result is a linking of the past with the present, the internal with the external. The therapist facilitates this linking foremost by maintaining the flow of the session and supporting the transitions between images. Verbal interpretation also makes conscious these links between a dramatic scene and the patients' other relationships. For example, the therapist offered a verbal interpretation near the end of this session when he pointed out members' concerns about how much he cared about the group. However, the drama therapist usually offers *action interpretations* by introducing new characters or variations in character that are shaped closely to the patients' internal, here-and-now, or external relationships. The therapist offered such an interpretation when he addressed Agnes in a whining voice as her child who hadn't visited. The scene was transformed according to the therapist's understanding of the meaning of the patients' dramatic role-playing. Agnes' energetic response indicated that the therapist was empathically in touch with her feelings. The result was a more conscious awareness in the group that they had angry feelings toward their children, and that these feelings were tolerable. The drama therapy session thus serves an important integrative function for group members by facilitating the linking among split-off areas of experience and by acting as midwife to the emergence and recognition of meaning in their interpersonal relationships.

II: Explorations in the Therapeutic Process

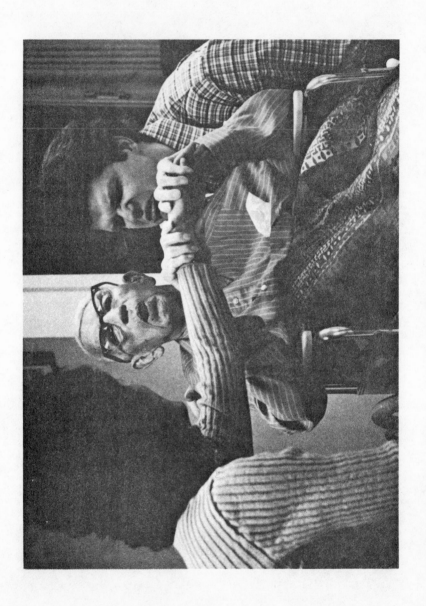

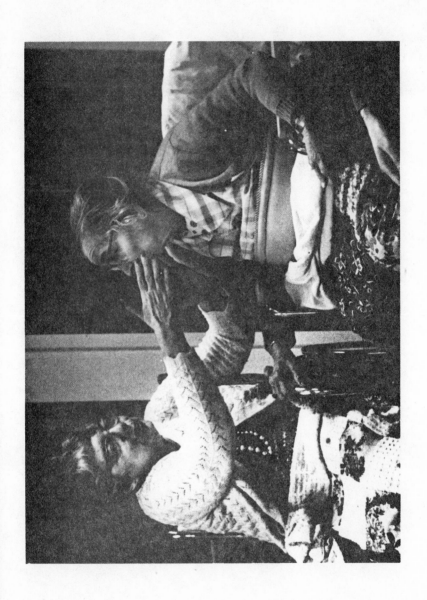

Chapter Six
Reminiscence in Movement Therapy

Susan L. Sandel

Several research studies have shown that reminiscing by the aged is an adaptational response and, as such, should be encouraged in the appropriate circumstances (Butler, 1963 and 1974; McMahon and Rhudick, 1967; Fallot, 1976; Lewis, 1971). I have found that group movement therapy offers an excellent opportunity for reminiscing, and that the therapist may utilize the reminiscences in developing peer interactions among the elderly. Reminiscing seems to encourage cognitive reorganization in confused or disoriented patients, as well as increasing self-esteem and socialization among all participants.

Reminiscence, the "act of thinking about or relating one's past experiences" (Webster's International Dictionary), is usually identified negatively with old age. Butler (1963) notes that reminiscing is commonly seen as hindering the older person's awareness of the present, and consequently is discouraged as a dysfunctional symptom of deterioration. However, life review, characterized by increased reminiscing, is a normal occurrence in older people. As Butler writes,

> . . . The life review is a naturally occurring, universal mental process characterized by the progressive return to consciousness of past experiences, and particularly, the resurgence of unresolved conflicts; simultaneously, and normally, these revived experiences and conflicts can be surveyed and reintegrated (p. 66).

Butler further suggests that the life review process which has been

Originally published as "Reminiscence in Movement Therapy With the Aged," *The Arts in Psychotherapy* (1978), Vol. 5, No. 4, 217-221. Reprinted by permission of ANKHO International, Inc.

stimulated by the awareness of impending death "potentially proceeds towards personality reorganization."

A study conducted by McMahon and Rhudick (1967) confirms
Butler's clinical findings that reminiscing is an adaptational
response. The investigators report:

> Reminiscing. . .is positively correlated with successful adap-
> tation to old age and appears to foster adaptation through main-
> taining self-esteem, reaffirming a sense of identity, working
> through and mastering personal losses, and contributing posi-
> tively to society (p. 78).

Their study also revealed that the group of subjects who were found
to be clinically depressed reminisced less than the nondepressed
group and showed greater difficulty in reminiscing. Similarly, Fallot's research (1976) substantiates the notion that reminiscing serves
an adaptive function in adulthood. This study also demonstrated the
direct role that reminiscing can play in lowering depressive affect.
One of the therapeutic implications of this work is that clinicians and
family members should attach more significance to reminiscing and
provide more opportunities for its legitimate expression.

MOVEMENT THERAPY STIMULATES REMINISCING

Movement therapy sessions with the elderly provide one arena
where reminiscing can be fostered in a purposeful manner and within a social context. In movement therapy sessions, the action is a
vehicle for interaction: that is, the primary focus is on how the
group responds to the opportunity for expressing feelings and socializing. This approach to movement therapy, based on dance therapy
techniques that were originally developed with psychiatric patients
(Chace, 1975), falls within the range of supportive approaches to
geriatric psychotherapy in which the therapist plays a relatively active role (Rechtschaffen, 1959).

Sessions begin with everyone sitting in a circle, with most patients in wheelchairs. Initially music is important for providing a
group rhythm, but may not be necessary for the entire session.
Warm-up exercises, which may be led by the patients themselves,
are conducive to images which are developed into interaction se-
quences. The movements stimulate associations and images which

one can use to facilitate patients verbalizing their memories. For example, in one group in a nursing home, the participants were all stretching their arms toward the center of the circle and pulling them back to their chests repeatedly. I asked, "What could we pull?" One client answered, "A rope on a boat." As we continued moving together, I asked if anyone in the group had ever been on a boat. Several people replied affirmatively, and a group discussion followed about the various boating and canoeing excursions that people had enjoyed as long ago as seventy years.

This progression from the sensory experience to a symbolic one and finally to a verbal level permits a spontaneous unfolding of material during the session. The therapist need not arbitrarily introduce a topic for the group, but can pick up on the issue suggested by the actual movements and images.

REORGANIZATION AND SOCIALIZATION

When participating in movements that remind them of past mastery experiences, confused patients often appear more alert and organized. The reminiscing seems to stimulate immediate, if short-lived, cognitive reorganization. One art therapist who gives assignments that encourage reminiscing has similarly observed that the old function better when they remember their younger, better functioning selves (Dewdney, 1973). Hellebrandt (1978) noted that senile dementia patients who did not respond to reality orientation did participate in a group activity involving reminiscing. When these patients were given notebooks entitled "This Is My Life," Hellebrandt observed, "it seemed remarkable that so much background material could be extracted from individuals who rarely if ever spoke spontaneously."

The following example is from a movement therapy session at the Sound View Specialized Care Center with five long-term female residents between the ages of 78 and 92. Admitting mental status exams revealed that four out of the five were confused, while three of the patients had diagnoses of organic brain syndrome. All of these women experienced extensive periods of confusion, and several did not know where they were until they entered the therapy room. Three of them participated minimally in verbal conversations, while one had lengthy spells of total muteness. All had been attending the movement therapy group weekly for at least six months.

DEVELOPMENT OF THE POTATO IMAGE

We were lifting our arms up and down slowly as part of the warm-up movements. I suggested that we raise our arms as if we were lifting something very heavy. I then suggested that we pass the heavy object around the circle from one person to the next. I asked, "What can we pass?" Ms. D. said, "A sack of potatoes." As we continued moving, Ms. D., who had grown up on a farm in Ireland, started telling the group all about potato farming. She detailed the process of planting potatoes, digging them up, storing them in the barn covered with hay, etc. I then asked, "What else could we do with the potatoes?" Ms. S. started throwing imaginary potatoes across the circle, which was picked up by the rest of the group with much laughter, including Ms. K., who had been mute until then.

I asked if we could do anything else with the potatoes; someone else suggested mashing them. Everyone then proceeded to "mash" the potatoes, with several people offering ingredients such as butter and salt, and giving directions concerning the proper way to prepare them. When I asked what we could do next, Ms. S. said gleefully, "Eat them!" and the women began "feeding" the mashed potatoes to one another. Discussion followed.

Ms. K: I'm a good cook. I can make soup.
Ms. Sc: I used to like to cook.
Therapist: Did anyone else like to. cook?
Ms. C: I was a good cook once.
Ms. S: (Turning to Ms. C., her roommate) M., you never told me you cook! (She looked respectfully at Ms. C.)
Ms. D: I did a lot of cooking. You know I have nine children. I used to like to feed them spinach in the winter; it was good for them.
Therapist: What else did you feed them?
Ms. D: I baked pies. Apple pies, with potato in the crust.
The conversation then shifted to a current concern—the food in the nursing home.
Ms. S: They gave us apples today—apples in a dish. It's not real apple pie (paused, looked around and made a face) I ate it anyway! (Big smile)

The group responded with giggles and nods.

Of significance is that these five women, supported by the structure of the movements and periodic interventions by the therapist, could sustain a logical sequence of cognitive and motor activity which lasted for 20 minutes. Even the less verbal patients contributed to a conversation organized around the memory of past competencies. Ms. S.'s regard for her roommate clearly increased when she learned that Ms. C. had been a good cook. Repeatedly, in such situations, patients learn about each other's accomplishments for the first time. The resulting interaction, occuring within the structured group experience, can be a first step toward socialization for patients who have been socially isolated.

EXPRESSION OF NEGATIVE AFFECT

Reminiscing in the movement therapy sessions is not always linked to positive experiences; it can also facilitate the verbalization of painful memories. In many institutions there are few opportunities for aged residents to express negative affect in a constructive way. Since angry outbursts and abusive language are abhorred by most residents and staff alike, many patients fear that they would be viewed as "impolite" or "ungrateful" if they openly expressed their negative feelings or critical attitudes. The intimacy that evolves in small movement therapy groups through sharing memories creates an atmosphere in which upsetting feelings and complaints may be aired. In a more alert group of seven residents ranging from 77 to 95 years old, the first expression of negative affect occurred after the group had been meeting weekly for nine months. The following took place in this group during the fourteenth month of the group's life.

Each individual took turns leading warm-up exercises which included a variety of hand movements such as talking to others with our hands. While we were doing this, there was talk of sickness (many residents had the flu) which developed into a symbolic group exercise of throwing away and pushing away sickness from the members of the group.

Mr. J.: Push it away; pull it back.
Mr. L: Why the hell do you want to pull it back?
Mr. J: Okay, push it away and leave it there!

I then suggested that we extend the movement so that we were rocking forward and back in our chairs. One woman mentioned that it

was an awful feeling to fall, and recounted an incident in which sh̬
had taken a bad fall. I asked if anyone else remembered falling. Mr.
J. remembered going ice skating and falling backwards on the ice.
Ms. K. and Mr. L. both shared their memories of breaking an arm
in a fall.

Ms. B: I don't remember falling. I was always very careful.
Mr. J: (In a joking tone) You're a fallen woman!
Ms. B: I should hope not (laughing). That would be something,
    wouldn't it!
(Everyone laughed, conversed, with neighbors.)

What is important here is not only the specific content of what
was discussed, but also the fact that people were able to share
unpleasant memories while maintaining a sense of humor in a spontaneous and largely unself-conscious manner. The reminiscences
developed from the sensorimotor experiences and provided a focus
around which the interaction occurred.

In another group of confused patients, we were exercising our
legs by lifting one foot after the other.

Mr. H: This reminds me of marching.
Ms. G: Aren't we too old to march anymore?
Ms. F: No.
Therapist: Did anyone ever march in a parade or a procession?
Mr. H: In the army. (He sings, "When the Caissons Go Marching
    Along," and several people join him.)
Therapist: (The group continued stamping their feet.) Anyone else
    ever march in a procession?
Ms. M: I know I have, but I can't remember. Maybe in school, yes
    school.
Therapist: Perhaps in a graduation procession?
Ms. M: Yes, that's it.
Ms. V: There were processions in Italy when Hitler came to power.
    All the soldiers marched down the streets. And processions for
    Mussolini.
Therapist: Can we march like soldiers? (The group responded with
    louder, more militant stamping.)
Ms. V: And then there were processions in Israel for the Jews who

were killed by Hitler. (She started to cry.) Many of my people
were killed there, in Europe.
(A co-therapist and patient on either side of her extended their hands
to her, as the rest of the group stopped stamping.)
Co-therapist: It's understandable that you feel sad about that.
Ms. V: I'm sorry to trouble you with my problems. They say I talk
too much.
Co-therapist: Who says that?
Ms. V: They all do.
Ms. S: We like hearing your stories.
Therapist: It's okay to tell us.
Ms. V: Thank you.

Although the reminiscence was not fully explored at that time, the
value that painful memories can be shared and that group members
are willing to listen was supported by the group. Despite the impact
of Ms. V.'s associations, the group did not fall apart, and Ms. V.
seemed much relieved when her pain was openly acknowledged.

REMINISCING LEADS TO HERE-AND-NOW INTERACTIONS

The reminiscing which develops from the action in movement
therapy sessions can lead to discussion about current issues in the
patients' lives. The activity itself and the memories which are
stimulated by it can be used by the therapist to facilitate here-and-
now interactions.

In the following episode, which occurred in the same group, a
massage exercise provoked memories of better days which, in turn,
evolved into a discussion of people's ages, physical limitations, and
past sexual activity.

Warm-up exercises involving patting our bodies developed into a
"group massage" in which staff and patients who could do so gently
massaged another person's shoulders. Several patients remembered
that years ago a nightly backrub was a regular part of the routine in
nursing homes. Ms. K. remarked that sometimes if you got the right
person to help you to bed, he or she would rub your back, but you
had to ask. The point was made by several people that one has to ask
for things nowadays, whereas in the "good old days" you got more
for your money.

After the massage, two patients stood up to dance, while the rest clapped and moved to the music in their wheelchairs. Ms. B. noted that she couldn't stand up, but that her roommate, Ms. V., could.

Ms. B: You're in good shape, Ms. V.

Ms. V: (Giggles.)

Ms. K: Better than most of us. I can't move my leg at all these days, and my brace needs to be fixed.

Ms. K. launched into a lengthy series of complaints about her paralyzed side and the problems with her braces, for which she received a great deal of sympathy from others.

Ms. J: Thank God I have no problems seeing or hearing!

Ms. G: I've got everything wrong with me. I can't see, I can't hear, and I've got arthritis.

Mr. J: I have problems with my eyes, too. (Turning to Ms. G.) After all, you're no 18-year-old anymore. How old are you, anyway?

Several people repeated the question for Ms. G. who had not heard all of it, and helped her calculate her age. Mr. J., who is 87, thought that Ms. G. looked older than he and was surprised to learn that she was a few years younger. At this point there was some joking about ages, especially with Ms. J. who has consistently refused to divulge her age, even on her birthday.

Therapist: Anyone else have other kinds of problems?

Mr. L: No problems (but pointed to his genitals emphatically and looked around).

Ms. B. saw this and gasped.

Mr. J: We see that you're the youngest in spirit around this place! Well, I think I'll start asking the nurses to give me back rubs at night. (He and Mr. L. exchanged winks and nods.)

The individuals in this group are just beginning to feel more comfortable expressing their concerns such as sexual frustration and loneliness. The physical contact, imagery, and reminiscing in the movement therapy sessions provide a supportive framework within which people can explore issues which many of them have not shared with others for many years.

DISCUSSION

Reminiscing, as it occurs within movement therapy sessions with the aged, appears to stimulate short-term cognitive reorganization among disoriented patients and socialization among patients with a wide range of physical and mental disabilities. Movement therapy is especially conducive to reminiscing which emerges spontaneously as a result of the sensory experiences; even the most disorganized patients may share in another's memory, if only on the physical level.

An important influence upon the atmosphere of these groups is the element of play which is inherent in the medium of movement and dance. This pervasive playfulness permits the participants to distance themselves, if necessary, from the seriousness of the content they may be offering. This type of approach seems to facilitate sharing and socializing among the aged, as Linden (1953) notes in his work with institutionalized women in which he encourages every opportunity for fun and laughter. I share the enthusiasm of other clinicians and researchers who have discovered that the aging respond positively to opportunities for recalling the past in a supportive setting. My own work and the observations of the other clinicians cited in this paper suggest that action-oriented groups which encourage reminiscing can provide an arena for social communication, particularly for those people who do not respond to other treatment modalities.

Chapter Seven
Exploring Sexual Issues Through Movement Therapy

Susan L. Sandel

The idea that sexual contact may have life-prolonging or invigorating effects is an ancient one found in several cultures. Such sexual contact does not necessarily refer to sexual intercourse, particularly among the aged, but rather the beneficial effects of physical contact, warmth, and intimacy. For example, the story of King David described the revitalization of the king resulting from the proximity of a young Shunammite woman who was brought to sleep in his bed in order that "the king may get heat" (1 Kings 1:2). This phenomenon, called gerocomy or Shunammitism, refers to the beneficial effects of a young woman's heat or breath on an older male. Verwoerdt (1976) likened this phenomenon to the current situation in nursing homes where young, usually female staff feed, bathe, and dress elderly patients. He speculated that the closeness experienced through the touching involved in caring for and feeding the older person may have restorative or regenerative effects in its sublimated form.

Unfortunately, many aged people are placed in situations which do not tolerate any form of sexual expression. Several research studies (Berezin, 1969; Butler & Lewis, 1973; Verwoerdt, 1976) have shown that although the incidence of actual sexual activity may decline with age, sexual interest does not. Acknowledging such interest may be beneficial in itself to the elderly when it stimulates a sense of vitality (Linden, 1955; Verwoerdt, 1976). Linden (1953) believed that neglecting the possibility of a sexualized transference

Originally published as "Sexual Issues in Movement Therapy With Geriatric Patients," *American Journal of Dance Therapy* (1979), Vol. 3, 4-14. Reprinted by permission of the American Dance Therapy Association.

between the therapist and client or ignoring memories of adult sexuality may deprive the older person of therapeutic opportunities. Such attitudes also diminish the aged person's feelings of self-respect and participation in an important aspect of human functioning. Group movement therapy sessions in which mutual touching, the expression of memories, and the sharing of feelings are encouraged, provide one place where nursing home residents may explore their sexuality.

The type of movement therapy described in this paper incorporates a flow of activity, development of group images, and relatively active therapist participation (Chace, 1975). The action is a vehicle for interaction which ideally unfolds in a supportive and accepting environment. The sound and movement activities in the movement therapy sessions sometimes create an atmosphere of excitement which may culminate in a "group catharsis," pairing among members, or conversation about sexual issues. For example, in one group of nursing home residents, ages 77-98, the holding of hands in a circle developed into a rigorous hand-shaking sequence. This was accompanied by the Beatles song, "I Wanna Hold Your Hand." A rythmic chant emerged in unison and excitement increased as the participants moved their arms up and down while looking at each other. The chant became a series of grunts, ending in a soft "aaah" sound. This sequence, which had an "orgasmic" quality, was followed by several people dancing in pairs, talking about choosing partners, and reminiscing about dancing in the past. For fifteen minutes there was sustained involvement and animated activity among people who are usually inert and isolated.

UTILIZING THE TRANSFERENCE

An important goal of movement therapy is to facilitate social interaction and peer involvement, a process which may also include the reawakening of dormant sexual interests. As the group members begin to view the therapist as a significant authority figure and transference object, the therapist may use individual transferences to further the development of a group identity. In this author's experience, initially the therapist is the recipient of the clients' erotic fantasies, jokes, and inquiries. Sometimes this takes a long time to happen.

For example, one group of elderly residents met for more than a year before they used my name, asked questions about my life, and wondered about my relationships outside the group. After I returned from a conference in California, one male participant asked if I had "just gone to meetings?" When I replied that I had seen a movie there, he playfully chided me in the group, saying that "I wasn't supposed to have a good time." A co-therapist reported that while I was absent there had been speculation about whether I would come back married.

This exchange and other similar conversations occurred around the time that there was an observable increase in peer interaction in this particular group (Kelleher, 1978). As Linden (1953) noted in his group psychotherapy sessions with senile women, ". . .the therapist can stimulate a good deal of rivalry among the members, become the target for a number of individual transferences, and by eventually shedding these allow identifications and group identity to take place" (p. 158). The resulting "lacework of transferences" becomes the vehicle for empathic identification among group members, which, in turn, creates a network of socialization.

The following example is from the same group of nursing home residents mentioned above. A simple gesture stimulated a group discussion in which the focus changed from individual dialogues with the therapist to spontaneous peer interaction.

The group sat in a circle, rocking from side to side and holding hands. Our motions changed from forward and backward rocking to gestures of opening and closing. As people wrapped their arms around themselves, I suggested that we give ourselves a pat on the back.

Therapist: Give yourself a nice big hug.
Mr. J.: I love myself.
Therapist: Every once in a while everyone needs a pat on the back.
Mr. L.: [To therapist teasingly] Hey, you're patting your arm!
Therapist: Is it a good feeling to love yourself?
Ms. K.: Sure. If you don't do it, who will?
Therapist: If you don't do it, who will, huh?

Mr. J.: [Laughingly] If you don't love yourself, nobody else will love you.

Therapist: Do you think that's so?

Mr. B.: You could get conceited if you do it yourself.

Therapist: If you love yourself too much?

Ms. B.: [Emphatically] Yes! That's not nice.

Mr. J.: No, it's not nice.

Ms. B.: It's not polite, is it?

Mr. J.: [Nods affirmatively.]

Therapist: What's the difference between loving yourself enough to feel good about yourself versus being conceited?

Ms. B.: I don't know.

Mr. L.: There's no difference. If you love yourself, have a big crush on yourself, it's just as bad as. . .

Ms. B.: Then you're vain.

Mr. L.: Yes, that's right. [To the therapist] You don't see it, huh?

Therapist: I was just wondering. Ms. K. was saying that it's important to like yourself in order for other people to like you.

Ms. K.: Well, *I* think so.

Ms. B.: If you don't like yourself, nobody else will. [Several people laugh.]

Therapist: What's the difference between that and being vain?

Ms. K.: A lot of difference. [Impatiently] It depends upon the circumstances.

Ms. B.: I see people come in my room, look in my mirror, fussing with their hair. That's vain.

Ms. K.: We all know the difference. It's up to us to know.

Mr. J.: We're all beyond that stage now. [People looking thoughtful.]

Mr. L.: [To therapist] That means you too! You're no exception! [Laughter]

Ms. K.: Come on now, Clyde.

Mr. L.: Well, you wouldn't make her an exception, would you?

Ms. K.: No, but I don't think you mean it the way I do! [There was a moment of silence.]

Mr. L.: [Softly] Well, I mean it. . . the honest way. [Turning] You're all right, Sue.

Ms. B.: [Turning to her neighbor] You're all right, Bea. There's nothing the matter with you.

[Everyone speaks simultaneously, turning to the people next to them.]

"You're all right."

"We're nothing for someone to go wild about, but we're all right I guess."

"You're okay."

SEXUAL BEHAVIOR

Geriatric clients in institutions sometimes express their rage, despair, or neediness through provocative sexual behavior. Overtly sexual provocativeness may mask underlying issues such as fears about losing control or concerns about physical deterioration. In psychologically unsophisticated facilities, disruptive behavior may be simply labeled a "management problem" and treated with medication or physical restraint. More subtle acting out, such as occasional exhibitionism or sexual overtures to staff, may even be considered "cute" in a very old person and subsequently ignored or benignly tolerated. Important communications may be overlooked if such behavior is not regarded as potentially meaningful to an individual.

Case Example

One 77-year-old male participant in a movement therapy group, Mr. L., frequently pinched female staff and had become increasingly interested in me and my co-therapist. When female visitors attended our movement therapy group, he would often assert leadership and become openly competitive with another male patient. He usually started the group by doing vigorous exercises, demanding that others follow him. Occasionally when Mr. L. sat next to me, he would hold my hand very tightly and try to "accidentally" brush his hand against my breast or shoulder. I responded to these advances by defining our territory through gentle nonverbal indications of the limits of our spatial boundaries within the context of the particular exercise. He would generally nod and smile mischievously at me.

Mr. L. seemed to have difficulty remembering the time of the group despite the co-therapist's reminders a few hours before. On a few occasions, he arrived at the movement therapy room more than one hour before the group was scheduled. Upon seeing that the room was empty, he would go to bed, angrily telling us later that *he* had been ready and no one else was there. More often, immediately after lunch, he would remove his clothes and go back to bed. He would then have to get up and dress himself again for the group. As he was a stroke victim, this was a slow and painful process for him. He would usually complain about having to endure this inconvenience, implying that he was doing us a great favor by attending the group.

After many weeks of this ordeal, I happened to be walking by his room as he was struggling to get his foot into his pants. He beckoned me to help. I did so willingly and to my surprise saw that he was not wearing any underwear. When I asked him why, he said gruffly that it was "too much trouble." Upon discussing this with other staff, I learned that Mr. L. usually did not wear underwear to movement therapy and was often aided in dressing by my young female co-therapist or an older female volunteer.

Mr. L.'s behavior raised many questions: Did he really forget the time of the group or was he using it as an excuse for additional attention and as a way of exerting control? Did he not wear his underwear because it was truly difficult for him to put it on, or was he intentionally exhibiting himself? Should this pattern be permitted to continue or should it be changed? Should it be insisted that he wear his underwear? Should the implications of his behavior be ignored or should he be directly confronted with these questions?

At the time, it was thought that for the therapist to ignore the possibility that Mr. L. was deliberately exhibiting himself and to regard it as "routine care" would communicate denial of the sexual feelings he was apparently experiencing. On the other hand, reprimands or rigid rules about underwear would set a battle of wills and probably induce shame. Since control was clearly a concern for Mr. L., a battle would have ensued over the terms of his participation in the movement therapy group. He seemed to be constantly struggling to let the staff know that he came by choice, that his presence should be appreciated, and that he had a right to get what he wanted from the group. Making his attendance contingent on accepting the therapist's terms (primarily including being dressed on time and wearing underwear) would be demeaning to him. As Mr. L.'s sexual feelings were apparently stimulated in the movement therapy group, they should be dealt with there rather than in the privacy of his bedroom.

Thus the staff decided not to interfere with Mr. L.'s ritual, but rather, to become more removed from it. That is, the co-therapist and therapist no longer aided Mr. L. in his dressing. He dressed himself with help from the ward staff who usually attended to his self-care tasks. Mr. L. subsequently began to express his sexual interests and frustrations more openly in the movement therapy group. This suggests that indeed he was trying to deal with sexual issues in his ward behavior and these issues were then channeled into the group when contact was limited to that arena. For example, when people were discussing their physical problems in one session, Mr. L. pointed to his genitals and indicated that this was his problem. A few group members were able to engage Mr. L., who usually denied that he had any problems to share with the group, in a brief dialogue about feeling sexually frustrated.

In retrospect, the author realized that she was feeling extremely uncomfortable, and perhaps avoided dealing directly with the sexual provocation. Berezin (1969) suggested that one motivation for ignoring or avoiding the sexual expressions of old people is rooted in the classical oedipal reaction. He stated, "The oedipal child fiercely clings to his conviction that his parents do not indulge in sexual activity, that they are and must be sexless" (p. 132). This corroborates Meerloo's (1955) concept of a reverse transference, a phenomenon among therapists who work with the elderly due to the fact that they are mostly younger than the patients, themselves. The author's reluctance to confront Mr. L.'s exposed genitals may have resulted in part from her oedipal anxiety evoked by the situation. An alternative interpretation is that the author felt uneasy when faced with the helplessness of Mr. L. when he was trying to dress himself. The author, as therapist, preferred to cling to her image of Mr. L. as he presented himself in the group as a feisty, flirtatious character. The author realized that she wanted to maintain the myth of his potency which often vitalized the movement therapy group and instilled her with hope. The desire to see Mr. L. as a whole person and to minimize his handicaps was perhaps another motivation for avoiding the difficult dressing ordeal.

FEMALE LONGEVITY

Several studies (Butler & Lewis, 1973) have shown that for women, the availability of a sexually capable partner is a crucial determinant of their sexual functioning in later life. However, there are many older women without partners. The dearth of men is painfully apparent in convalescent homes where there are typically four times

more women than men. Even for the very aged residents, this issue
is a real concern and may emerge as a topic of discussion in the
movement therapy group. In many institutions, there are few structured opportunities for residents to express their feelings and
thoughts about such concerns. The intimacy that develops in small
movement therapy groups contributes to the creation of an atmosphere which supports the expression of otherwise taboo subjects.

In one group of seven women and one man, the following
dialogue occurred after the co-therapist announced that a former
female resident had been transferred to another facility and had
found a boyfriend. The protagonist in this discussion, Ms. B., is an
88-year-old, severly physically disabled woman who is confined to a
wheelchair and experiences periods of disorientation.

> *Ms. B.:* Yes, I like men, lots of men. There's not enough men
> around here—hardly any around. [Turning towards Mr. J.,
> the one man in the group] This poor man looks lonely all
> by himself. I wish I could go over and visit him sometimes.
> [She looks at him seductively, smiling.]
> *Therapist:* Do you ever visit him?
> *Ms. B.:* Oh no. I wouldn't have the nerve. Besides, Bea [her
> roommate] wouldn't let me. She's always watching me.
> She's a real eagle eye.
> *Ms. G.:* What's that? [The co-therapist repeated Ms. B's
> words for Ms. G. who is extremely hard of hearing.]
> *Ms. G.:* That's a hot one.
> *Co-Therapist:* How do you feel about that, Bea?
> *Ms. V. [Bea]:* If Marge wants to make friends with a man, I'd
> help her out.
> *Ms. B.:* I can't go anywhere without Bea. I'd be lost without
> her.
> *Mr. J.:* You can't live with her and you can't live without her.

Underneath the playful and often humorous exchange was the acknowledgement of Ms. B's longing for male companionship as well
as her extreme dependency upon her roommate. Her willingness to
banter about her dilemma evoked positive regard from the staff and
other clients who had previously equated her dependency with a lack
of interest in her environment and peers. Sometimes such issues
elicit dramatic responses from people who seem to be otherwise un-
responsive or even asleep. One 86-year-old woman succinctly

summed up this particular dilemma when she was asked how she spends her time in a convalescent home. She replied crisply, "I eat, sleep, and I'd f____ if I could find someone."

HUMANIZING THE ENVIRONMENT

Movement therapy provides one arena in the convalescent home where sexual issues may be acknowledged and explored. Even the most disorganized patients may respond lucidly when given the opportunity to deal with sexual concerns. Overt sexual behavior may have a potentially disruptive influence on institutional life and therapists must be aware of their own feelings and reactions. Ideally, the supportive atmosphere and spirit of playfulness in the movement therapy sessions facilitate dealing with these sexual issues, including painful or embarrassing material. Some patients have been surprisingly open in their discussions of sexual interest and limitations. This is especially true when the therapist establishes an attitude of serious regard, tempered by the warm atmosphere of the movement therapy session.

Although movement therapy offers no encompassing solutions for solving the sexual frustrations of the infirm aged, it does offer opportunities for structured physical contact, mutual caring, and open discussion. Touching and being touched appear to have a rejuvenating effect on the participants which increases their alertness and responsiveness to others. Movement therapy, by humanizing the environment, provides opportunities for geriatric patients to experience their sexuality more freely.

Chapter Eight
Insight and Transference
in Drama Therapy

David Read Johnson

BACKGROUND

This chapter will describe group psychotherapy with nursing home residents, ages 64-96, which utilizes the nonverbal and symbolic activities of drama therapy to facilitate an orientation to insight and transference phenomena.

Psychotherapy was initially considered to be of little value to the elderly, whose rigidity and interpersonal withdrawal supposedly interfered with the development of insight, and thus, personality change (Abraham, 1949; Freud, 1905/1962). Until the 1950's, few psychological interventions were considered appropriate for the very old. Since the 1950's, various forms of group therapy have been developed (Goldfarb, 1953; Oberleder, 1966; Schwartz and Goodman, 1952; Shere, 1964; Silver, 1950; Wolff, 1963). Many utilize supportive approaches in which the therapist plays an active and reassuring role, and socialization is the central goal. Discussion of painful life events, the effect of physical limitations, or dependency issues arising within the transference are typically avoided. The therapist's task, instead, is to facilitate reminiscence of positive memories, sharing of common concerns, and problem-solving.

The fact that many of these groups are effective need not be interpreted as evidence that the elderly cannot tolerate or benefit from insight-oriented approaches that might focus more directly on painful life events or transference phenomena. The factors responsible for the scarcity of expressive group psychotherapy with the elderly are not clear. Linden (1953) and Butler (1974) have described sev-

Originally published as "Expressive Group Therapy With the Elderly: A Drama Therapy Approach," *International Journal of Group Psychotherapy* (1985), Vol. 1, 109-127. Reprinted by permission of the American Group Psychotherapy Association, Inc.

eral culturally held myths about the elderly that may be responsible. These include (1) transference is not possible in senile patients, (2) the elderly lack the flexibility required for insight, and (3) the elderly should disengage from others to prepare for death.

Berland and Poggi (1979) have recently described a successful example of the expressive approach with aged patients 77-91 years, in a retirement home. They base their work on Linden's (1953, 1954, 1955, 1956) and Benaim's (1957) early appreciation of the role of transference and the ability to achieve insight among elderly patients. These authors found that their clients expressed desires to learn about themselves and to talk about painful issues that were disturbing them. The therapists then shifted from their initially more supportive stance. Transference interpretations by the therapists were utilized effectively by the patients, who, in more ways than not, acted like any other group therapy clients.

The innovative work reported by Berland and Poggi (1979) suggests that the ability to tolerate insight-oriented approaches to group therapy is not dependent upon age. However, this ability may be dependent upon relatively unimpaired cognition and the ability to communicate verbally. Berland and Poggi did screen their patients for such qualities, and one suspects that their sample would be among the higher functioning patients in most nursing homes. The ability to engage in relatively unstructured discussion and appreciate the level of abstraction in many transference and group process interpretations may be a determining factor in who will benefit from expressive psychotherapy, regardless of age (Yalom, 1975).

This chapter, which supports the contentions of Berland and Poggi, aims to show how expressive, insight-oriented group psychotherapy, using the symbolic and nonverbal medium of creative drama, can be extended to elderly patients whose cognition and ability to communicate verbally are impaired.

CREATIVE ARTS THERAPIES AND THE ELDERLY

The creative arts therapies have increasingly been used in the treatment of the elderly. Reports of art therapy (Crossin, 1976; Dewdney, 1973; Zeiger, 1976), dance therapy (Fersh, 1980; Garnet, 1972; Irwin, 1972), and drama therapy (Burger, 1981; Gray, 1974; Michaels, 1981; Shaw, 1980) have spanned the full range of age (50-100 years), setting (senior center to nursing home), and diagnosis (unimpaired, physically limited, psychiatric). Nearly all of these approaches are supportive, in which re-activation, socialization, and positive self-esteem are encouraged. The nonverbal media seems useful in stimulating patients' orientation, interaction, and reminiscence, particularly for those with verbal difficulties.

Berger and Berger (1973) describe a unique format in which a group of psychogeriatric outpatients met three times a week for three hours. The first hour was verbal group psychotherapy, followed by dance therapy and relaxation exercises. Although this group was prematurely ended, the patients showed signs of significant improvement.

DRAMA THERAPY

Drama therapy has particular relevance to communication in patients with impaired cognition since it utilizes developmentally earlier modes of representation (i.e., sensorimotor and symbolic) as well as abstract, lexical forms (Bruner, 1964). The contribution of the dramatic medium to the therapeutic process consists of three factors: concretization, simplification, and symbolization. First, in drama therapy, feeling states, memories, and preconscious thoughts are concretized in improvisational enactments, allowing communication ordinarily interfered with by impairment in verbal expression (Irwin, Baker and Bloom, 1976; Johnson, 1981b, 1982a; Schattner and Courtney, 1981). The physicalization of memories appears to increase the cueing of relevant verbal associations (Werner and Kaplan, 1964). Second, the interpersonal dimensions of improvisational drama in group therapy provide opportunities for patients to enact a variety of part-selves which are normally suppressed. The demands on the self for social propriety and integration in normal social interaction are temporarily suspended in improvisational role-playing, where more simplified and incomplete personality fragments are tolerated. At the same time, the participation as a group in this playful action serves to enhance group cohesion. Third, the creation of a "free play" environment establishes a transitional space in which reality and fantasy are temporarily, but safely, intermixed (Winnicott, 1953). The therapist and group members are given access to symbolizations of internal states, which later can be linked to past familial and current transferential conflicts through the use of interpretations. These three elements of drama therapy will be dem-

onstrated more fully in the following example of group psychotherapy with the elderly.

Case Example

The author has conducted a group at a private nursing home for
over four years. It is named the "Drama Therapy Group" and consists of 7-9 residents, aged 64-96 years (most are in their 80's), and
a co-therapist. The group meets once a week for an hour. The mental and physical condition of the group members varies, from mild
confusion to complete alertness, and from physical integrity to severe physical impairment. While most of the residents are expected
to arrive by themselves, several more impaired patients are brought
to the group by the therapists. Most of the patients are confined to
wheelchairs. The group has a closed membership. The therapists
evaluate referrals from nursing and recreation staff when a vacancy
occurs, usually due to a transfer of a resident to another nursing
home. The stated purpose of the group is often explained as "to get
to know each other and share your feelings with the group."

The therapists are warm, relatively active, and seek to establish a
playful atmosphere in the group. They are also quite confrontive
about residents' family problems, physical limitations, and transferential feelings about the therapists. For the therapists, the purposes
of the group are (1) to serve as an orienting and socializing environment, (2) to be an arena for sharing reminiscences about important
life events, and (3) to aid in the acceptance of one's physical limitations, interpersonal losses, and eventual death.

Structure of the Sessions

The sessions typically begin with free discussion until one of the
patients, or occasionally the therapist, initiates a ritual movement
warmup, in which each member leads the group in making a simple
repetitive motion with accompanying vocal sound (e.g., raising both
arms and saying "Ahh"). Each member takes turns. Very often,
spontaneous imagery emerges from these motions, which is then developed into short role-plays involving some family theme.

In one session, Fanny was leading a motion in which each person
thrust their hand forward and shouted "Ha!" This was spontaneously transformed to "Ahh, *Ha!*" and pointing a finger. The therapist
asked the group what this action reminded them of, and Lora

shouted, "Ah, ha, I've caught you!" The group then repeated this motion, only directing it toward each other, saying, "Ah, ha, I've caught you!" The therapist then instructed Lora to direct this action to the person on her right, Fanny, who was to respond spontaneously. Fanny responded by saying, "You've caught me with my hand in the cookie jar! I'm sorry, Mother." Then Fanny repeated the original motion and phrase to the person on her right, and so on around the circle. Each pair engaged in a short improvisation in which one party had "caught" the other. Typically, a mother-child scene developed in which the child had been caught doing something naughty. Often the group members used actual family situations from their past.

The remainder of the session is a mixture of improvisational role-playing and discussion. The role-plays increasingly integrate material from patients' memories and current perceptions of their families, the group, or the nursing home. The therapists support this move toward more personal and affect-laden topics. For example, in the session described above, concerns about sexual activity emerged. Group members discussed their various experiences hiding their sexual activity from their parents, and several role-playing situations were then acted out based on these memories. As the group's associations to this issue developed, the therapists were able to link them to the group's fantasies about the sexual activity of the male and female co-therapists. Thus the movement and imagery facilitate the organization and concretization of the group's associations, which lead to more explicit discussions of past family situations as well as the current transference situation in the group. The session typically ends with a unison chant of "Drama Group!," as everyone holds hands and raises them up together.

Phases of the Group's Development

Initially, the group members tested out the degree to which support and nurturance were provided by the group and the therapists. Requests to be brought to the group, or to have parties, alternated with attempts to go to the bathroom or to visit relatives during the session. Group members tried to view the group as a series of "games" and were hesitant to discuss personal problems. Fanny shouted, "Only pleasant things!" whenever a negatively-toned topic emerged. The potential threat of the group experience was often expressed in group stories, which were created by going around the circle and having each member contribute a sentence. One story, for example, began: "It is night and dark. It's nice by the fire. We are all together." Soon, however, a hound howls and threatens to eat them, causing the fire to get out of control. In the end, everyone flees and climbs their own tree. Other stories included being on a raft fighting off sharks, or hiding in a cave, snuggled up to a teddy bear who turns into a grizzly bear.

The therapists remained tolerant of these group-level fears. As familiarity and cohesion increased, however, the sense that the group had become a stable and secure environment was established. Evidence of this achievement was apparent when the disorientation of several more impaired patients decreased dramatically when they attended the group. Soon, desires to share more personal problems, coupled with fears of revealing themselves, emerged in the symbolic imagery of the dramas. Images of death, journeys into the unknown, burying and unburying, and abandonment foreshadowed the direct discussion of these issues in the group.

The expression of unconscious aggressive and threatening material through the dramatic medium seemed to facilitate the eventual direct expression of these concerns by the group members. Threatening material could be openly expressed but temporarily disowned if the patient was not yet ready to acknowledge it. One was "only acting." After several months, the group was able to move back and forth between metaphorical and direct expression of threatening subjects such as physical limitations, death, family conflicts, and feelings about the therapist. The therapist often facilitated this shift through interpretations of patients' behavior in the role-playing, while at the same time supporting and participating in the playful atmosphere it created. Three examples of this process will now be described.

1. *Confronting Physical Limitations.* Most of the group members suffered from some severe physical limitation (loss of hearing or sight, stroke, Parkinson's disease). The mere inclusion of movement in the group's activities forced recognition of many of these limitations early in the group's life. The therapists did not avoid mentioning these problems directly or try to design exercises in which certain members would not have to use an impaired limb. Rather, if the group took hands, and one member hesitated to hold Chauncey's paralysed hand which was in a brace, the therapist would say, "It's all right to hold Chauncey's hand, Lora. Chauncey has had a stroke which prevents him from feeling much in his hand,

but you won't hurt it.'' As soon as there was some evidence that a particular limitation was noticed in the group, the therapists directly identified it. Often the group gave a sympathetic response, to which the particular patient showed mild embarrassment and then relief. Other group members then shared something about their own limitations.

In a session two years into the group's life, the group was making a motion with their hands. Chauncey, attempting to shake his paralysed hand, became frustrated and said, ''Not much of a hand.''

> *Th*: What would you like to do with it?
> *Chauncey*: Get rid of it.
> *Th*: You know where we put things in this group which we want to get rid of.
> *Lenore*: The magic box—bring down the magic box!

The ''Magic Box'' is a pretend box which is kept in the ceiling above the group. It can be brought down at any point in the session. Once its lid is carefully pulled off, anything can be found in the magic box, and anything can be put into it. Initially, members used it to find things they wished for (e.g., money, health). However, the box became an important reservoir of important parts of group life—people, bad feelings, wishes, and prayers were all placed in the box. When the box was reexamined in subsequent weeks, these things were brought out again to see if any changes had occurred. Thus the Magic Box allowed the therapists to temporarily legitimize omnipotent, expulsive or idealistic defenses (i.e., getting rid of bad things, finding good things). The Magic Box becomes an impersonal container of these projections, and the therapist, by reopening and reexamining its contents, in effect makes an ''action interpretation.'' The following excerpt shows how the dramatic exercise is used to interpret members' overly wishful fantasies about the group and the therapist.

> The group held hands and gave their ritual chant (a hum), bringing the magic box down, and then unscrewed the lid.
> *Th*: Okay, let's go around and get rid of any part of your body that doesn't work right. You start, Chauncey. Say something to it as you throw it in.
> *Chauncey* (throwing in his ''hand''): You're not much good.
> *Leila*: I wish my legs would work so I could walk.

Lenore: (tearful) I'm throwing in my hysterectomy. I could have had kids except for you.

Alicia: I'm throwing in my loneliness. I'm lonely.

Th: But what part of your body is that, Alicia?

Alicia: I don't know. I guess my heart. It's broken.

John (smiling): I'm throwing in the part that doesn't work as well as it used to.

Th: What part is that?

John: The male part. (Laughter).

Lenore: Reverend! How could you!

Th: Look into the box—what do people see?

Chauncey: Lots of things—real mess, isn't it?

Bessie: Bag of bones.

Lenore: Well, David, are you going to fix it?

Th: You mean I'm supposed to fix all your broken limbs? Do I have that kind of power?

Leila: Yes, of course. (General agreement).

Lora: No, he doesn't. Only God can fix something like that.

Th: People seem to have a lot of hope that this group, and doctors in general can solve your problems.

This comment provoked a long and involved discussion about their feelings of disappointment and frustration with their medical doctors and the nursing home. Angry feelings about the drama therapy group were avoided. The therapist finally said:

Th: I guess we'll have to see whether this group is powerful enough to repair all our broken parts. Take a look into the box again. We'll give it our "Zap," and see if anything changes. Ready?

The group then in unison raised their hands and thrust them toward the center with a loud "Zap." Each member then in turn took back their body part and said whether it was fixed or not.

Chauncey: No, mine's the same. I guess I'll just have to get along without it. It gives me character, don't you think?

Lenore: It's too late for me to have kids anyway.

Lora: Only God can change my loneliness. He'll take me when he's ready.

John: Look, mine's all fixed. Better watch out girls!

The "Zap," like the Magic Box, evokes and channels the group's omnipotent fantasies about its own powers. Often by so outrageously enacting the omnipotent desire, group members see immediately that they have been harboring unrealistic wishes. Gratification of the desires occurs on the level of play, however, which frees up the ego to perform its reality testing functions. Concomitantly, the humor reduces the pressure from the superego: one is forgiven for having the omnipotent wish (Freud, 1927/1962; Levine, 1977).

Each member's style of coping with their severe physical limitations is evident in their last comments, which appear to be attempts to reassure themselves in response to harsh internal reproaches about their physical deterioration. Since most of their physical limitations are permanent or progressive, their level of awareness of them is linked to their methods of coping with hopelessness and the inevitability of their own death.

2. *Death of the Self: Death of the Parents.* Concerns over death usually emerged in rather explicit ways in the role-playing. The group spent many hours enacting rituals of throwing things away, burying objects, and even conducting funerals. In one session, they were eating pretzels which had been baked by another group. They did not like the pretzels. The group placed their pretzels in an ashtray in the middle of the group and covered them with a napkin. In a playful way, the group pretended to bury "the old pretzel," who is "no good for anything anymore." The therapist then wondered aloud if group members were ever concerned about how people would feel about them after their deaths. The group immediately discussed how many of their relatives would be relieved, say "good riddance," etc. Alicia tearfully spoke about how she felt like a "bag of nothing."

In another session, John, the reverend, whose health had been failing, discussed his feelings about death and his sadness in missing the group. The group decided that in order to preserve him, they would put him in the Magic Box "so we can bring you out for each session." The group began its chant. John, with a smile, gave a benediction and eulogy about himself, causing some laughter. The therapist suggested that the group seemed concerned about whether John would remember *them* after he was gone. John then pretended to "speak from the grave" and, again humorously, insulted most of the group members and especially the therapist. The members parried with jokes about forgetting John completely after all. The therapist then said that in addition to wondering about whether they will be remembered by loved ones after they die, they might also be concerned about whether the therapist would remember them next week on his vacation. Did he care for them, or like John, was he glad to be away from these stupid old people?

The group confirmed this in various ways. Lenore noted that the therapist had not sent them a postcard during his last vacation. Leila thought he had had enough of them and needed a rest. John wasn't "too impressed" with the way he had been leading the group recently. The group discussed whether they would meet alone without the therapist. Chauncey, in fact, said, "We can't let this group die just because *he's* not here."

Members' defenses in relation to their own deaths were far more intact in comparison to their tremendously ambivalent and unresolved feelings about their own parents' deaths. These particular losses, about which they felt especially helpless, had left them psychologically alone and had forced them to seek new objects for their dependency needs. In most cases, these new objects were their children. In the group therapy context, the therapist becomes the object of these ambivalent dependency needs, and, like their children, is alternatively imaged as the dependent child and the dependable parent.

The issue of their parents' deaths arose in one session as the group was moving together. Lenore was leading a motion with her hands which reminded the group of climbing a rope. The image then changed to a beanstalk. As the whole group proceeded to climb the stalk, the therapist asked, "Where are we going?" "To heaven," Fanny cried out. The group climbed up to heaven. The therapist then asked, "Who are we going to speak to? Who is up here?" Lenore replied, "My parents are up there. They died many years ago, and it was the worst time of my life. In one year they both died, and I was left alone." The therapist then said, "Here we are in heaven, and here they are (pointing to the center of the circle). What would you like to say to them?" Each member of the group then took turns talking to their parents. Some said very little, others engaged in sad and touching conversations. In two cases, the therapist portrayed one of their parents. Following these enactments, the group shared memories of their parents.

These powerful themes, of their own and their parents' deaths, fueled much of the symbolic enactment and transference to the therapist during the sessions. The therapist, like their parents, is a dependable protector and, like their children, will live on after them. He is therefore the parent who will not die, who has not died.

Maintenance of this transferential image of the therapist serves to protect members from the full force of their anxieties about death. The dynamics are similar to those fueling religious beliefs in God, who also is the parent who does not die.

Given the tremendous power of this image, it is not surprising that in groups with the elderly, direct, verbal discussions of death are often characterized by an attitude of pseudo-acceptance, consisting of "God will take me when He's ready." The playful medium of drama seems to offer an acceptable vehicle for the more aggressive, mocking, and illicit feelings associated with death to be expressed, without threatening the integrity of the therapist's image. This was apparent in the grave scene where the group tolerated humorous attacks on the group members and the therapist.

3. *Transference to the Therapist*. Meerloo (1955) and Linden (1955) have noted that the transference with the elderly is a unique mixture of therapist-as-parent and therapist-as-child. The author's understanding of the transference situation with many nursing home patients is as follows: By the time a person becomes a patient in a nursing home, he is usually dependent upon his children or others of the next generation. Previously he had been the caregiver for his children, and often his parents in their advanced years as well. Now, his parents have gone and his children have taken the parental role toward him. Parent and child have traded places out of necessity, yet this reversal of the relationship is often a highly ambivalent one, entailing some embarrassment and resentment of the children. The therapist becomes both the object of idealization as the magical replacement of the loving and dependable parent and, at the same time, the resented child who has usurped the parental role.

The therapist's role in society supports the first representation, while the therapist's younger age supports the latter. Nevertheless, these two basic transference positions often conflict. Expression of the envy or resentment toward the therapist-as-child might threaten the image of the therapist-as-parent, so these feelings are repressed or more often displaced onto nursing staff or other patients. However, subtle put-downs, mocking, and teasing of the therapist often emerge. The therapist feels he is being treated like a child one moment, and overly idealized the next. Fear that their hostility or resentment will emerge stimulates the patients to increase their helpless behavior in the group so as to insure the maintenance of the dependable parental image.

This transference situation mirrors the actual situation between the patient and his/her own children, who often have taken over the decision-making and parental functions in the extended family. Many patients suppress their feelings of rage at the children for placing them in the nursing home, out of fear that they will no longer visit or write. Thus their helpless and dependent behavior serves both to keep the family engaged and to punish them.

The desire for an outlet for these feelings is particularly strong among many patients. This becomes evident when the therapist plays the child of the patients in the role-playing: tremendous affect is evoked. The resentment, hostility, and humiliation is able to find expression without threatening the image of the therapist, since he is only "playing." Once the scene is played, however, the therapist and the observing egos of the patients can more easily identify and acknowledge the existence of these feelings.

The therapist can initiate a role-playing often by simply addressing in a whiney manner one of the patients as "Mother!" or "Dad!," provoking much advice-giving, attempts at discipline, and furious arguments over him. After the role-playing, the group usually feels compelled to discuss how this particular child is similar or dissimilar to their own. Striking improvements in patients' orientation, reasoning, and verbal fluency frequently occur in these role-plays, presumably due to the relevance and power of these specific issues.

In the role-playing, the therapist and the female co-therapist are often paired as the young and naive couple who need guidance from their parents (played by the patients). In one session, Bessie initiated a rocking motion, which the group suggested was "rocking a baby carriage." From this image a role-play began in which the two therapists were married and about to have a child. They were talking to their parents, aunt and uncle about their feelings and need for advice. The group was very involved, arguing about how to have the child, the role of the father, and what its name should be. Lora suddenly pointed to the female therapist and said she looked awfully "big." Soon the mother was in labor and the child was given birth by its grandparents (played by two patients). The therapists sat rocking the (pretend) baby. Fanny suggested the baby be named "Drama Group." The baby was then passed around the group, so each member could say something to it. To the therapists' surprise, the baby was poked, dropped, insulted, and criticized by the patients, albeit in a humorous way. The therapists took the baby back.

As the therapists sat rocking the group's baby, the spontaneity in the group dropped noticeably. The therapist then commented that members seemed jealous of the baby, as if it was getting more attention and care from the therapists than they were. An awkward silence followed. The therapist then commented that even though it might seem strange to be envious of the therapists' pretend baby, he could understand it, since they had lost their own parents, who had taken care of them. At this point, Lenore and Fanny began crying, saying that they missed their parents and that they felt alone. Lora said how humiliating it was to be like a child to one's own children—it was better not to bother them. The group continued to share their feelings of loss and their sense of embarrassment about seeming so helpless in front of the (much younger) therapists. The therapists acknowledged that the group indeed had strong feelings about them, which seemed inexplicable to the group.

The key traumatic event in the lives of these patients is not their own deaths, which are to come, but the event that initiated the transfer of dependency upon their children—the death of their parents. This event is obviously represented in the transference as alternating images of the therapist as parent and as child. The therapists' resistance to seeing the importance of this event, especially in light of how unresolved patients' feelings about it are, is worthy of greater attention.

Countertransference with the Elderly

The initial phase of the group's existence was characterized by group members' collective stance against meaningful personal involvement with each other. The therapist's unconscious collusion with this was based on a romantic vision, shared by the wider culture, that each elderly person has embarked on a lonely journey towards death, necessitating their withdrawal from others in the world about them. Expression of their tremendous dependency needs and omnipotent wishes was justified (and therefore contained) by this defensive, heroic myth. Thus the therapist unconsciously responded to the group in terms of his own internal image of the heroic Self facing Death. This countertransferential attitude, shared culturally, may be one reason why most group therapies with the elderly have been supportive.

Once the drama therapy group had established itself over several months, and the therapist had helped to create an atmosphere of consistency, stability, and security, the defenses against intimacy (in both patients and the therapist) diminished. The group was now clearly important to its members, and it was more difficult to maintain the image of each member in an independent struggle with Death. Patients and therapist were more clearly in struggles with each other.

The full force of dependency issues and wishful fantasies broke through in the group as group members began to reinvest in interpersonal relationships. Each attempt at reinvestment, however, evoked memories of another loss. Each patient had in fact lost many loved ones. These losses stimulated equally intense searches for replacements, reenactments, and re-creations of past relationships. The intense reminiscing which occurred at this time represented preparation for reinvestment in new relationships as much as letting go of old ones.

The therapist, as a central figure in the group, became the focus of patients' efforts to relive the past. They often did this by comparing him to their own children or themselves when they were children, or merely by treating him like a child. The therapist, more familiar with transference situations in which he was a parental presence, initially misunderstood the group's effort to turn him into their child, and he resisted it. On one level the therapist's own struggles to be treated as an adult by his parents were evoked. He also may have been dimly aware of the ludicrousness of someone nearly one-third the age of the group members being seen as the wise and beneficent father. Being treated as young and less mature than the group was therefore most unbearable because it was true. The therapist was also vulnerable to anxieties aroused by being a child burdened with the task of caring for his parents, on whom he would prefer to depend.

The therapist's struggle against this reverse transference to the elderly serves to maintain the patients in a dependent, childlike role. The therapist's unconscious resistance sacrifices a preferable therapeutic neutrality (i.e., remaining psychologically equidistant from the specific projections as parent or as child). At a deeper level, however, the therapist's resistance is motivated by his own fear of death. As the parent to these elderly people, who need his assistance in facing death, he remains beyond death—the parent who does not die. The group colludes in this effort in order to cushion or deny the loss of their own parents. The therapist and group join together in this way to conquer death. If the therapist is seen for who he is, a child of older parents, then he too enters the progressive, multi-generational life cycle, which ends in death. Thus, psychologically, the group attempts to sustain the therapist as a representation of immortality.

The force which functions against this trend, aside from reality, is the patients' sense of humiliation in being treated as children by their children and their rage at this usurpation. The therapist experiences this feeling of humiliation when patients feel comfortable enough to chide him about his age or treat him as a child.

It is critically important for the therapist to be able to tolerate the transferential identification as a child. When the author recognized his own defensive stance, the group responded with greater spontaneity and involvement. Structuring the role of the child in role-playing, when the therapist actually "played" the patients' children or parents, introduced a useful separation between alternate transferential images of the therapist. Humiliating attacks on the therapist-as-child in the role-playing did not overly disrupt the protective, parental image usually maintained by group members.

SUMMARY

This chapter has attempted to describe the structure and process of a drama therapy approach to group psychotherapy with the elderly. Consistent with Berland and Poggi (1979) and Linden (1953), it was found that the elderly are capable of confronting and developing insight into anxiety-laden issues. The nonverbal and symbolic medium of movement and drama facilitate this process in three ways: (1) By creating a playful and metaphorical atmosphere, conflictual material is expressed more easily since, if necessary, it can be more easily disowned. The need for patients' anxieties to be denied, displaced, or to remain unexpressed is diminished. (2) The role-playing and physical movement concretize and simplify complex feeling states, increasing group members' ability to focus on a limited aspect of psychic or interpersonal experience. By evoking associations from kinesthetic and symbolic spheres, their cognitive resources are extended beyond abstract, verbal reasoning. (3) The group situation stimulates intense searches for replacements, reminiscences, and reenactments of relationships with lost loved ones. Dramatic role-playing, where in fact lost husbands, parents, and children are recreated by other group members, contributes to the reinvestment in other people as vehicles for meaningful relationships.

Group members became strongly invested in this group, and were quite active in other nursing home activities. The death rate in this group was one-third that of the nursing home at large, though no controlled study has been conducted. Groups of this type can have a major impact on the atmosphere of the nursing home, increasing the sense of spontaneity, hopefulness, and life, through the development of meaningful interpersonal relationships.

Chapter Nine
Expressive Group Therapy
with Severely Confused Patients

Susan L. Sandel

Music and movement are now recognized as activities of choice for people with various types of senile dementia, including Alzheimer's Disease (Caplow-Lindner et al., 1979; Needler & Baer, 1982). Sense memories are activated that, in turn, stimulate reminiscing and interaction. The modes of music and body action are vehicles through which the therapist makes contact with clients in the sensorimotor sphere. These activities, when conducted in an atmosphere of acceptance and sociability, help maintain and even improve a regressed individual's social functioning, particularly for previously isolated people. Consistency in time, place, group membership and activities contribute to the establishment of a safe and familiar environment in which even very confused people can participate and form links with others (Chapter 2). Rituals, such as singing games, group cheers, and repetitive movements provide modes of communication for those who have lost their communicative skills.

Groups of well and alert elderly are typically able to develop a sense of a group identity. Participants continuously adjust their own behavior to correspond to the values, goals, and norms of the group. For example, in one group with alert elderly in a nursing home, the members are cognizant of the time and place of the group meeting. Those who are ambulatory assist others in getting to the room in their wheelchairs; upon arriving, they arrange themselves in a circle. Most people know one another's names, or at least recognize the group members by sight. They chat until the therapist arrives, at which time they immediately begin a sound and movement exercise that involves taking turns with the leadership (Chapter 5). In this group, the values, norms and structures have been internalized by the participants. The elements of space (circle), task (warm-up exercise), and role (sharing leadership) are embedded in the group members' expectations and behaviors. Initially, a group is dependent upon the therapist for instruction, guidance, and modeling. In time, as structures become familiar and are internalized, the group proceeds with minimal verbal reminders from the therapist.

In movement therapy groups with severely confused elderly, on the other hand, the therapist is challenged to make contact with isolated individuals for whom a shared notion of a group does not exist. Since the therapist alone is able to maintain the notion of a group, s/he is the primary link among the participants, as well as the major tie to social reality. In a previous paper, the author has defined this phenomenon as the *nascent group*:

> An outstanding characteristic of the nascent group is that, while the group as an integrated and differentiated pattern of interaction among members does not objectively exist, it does exist phenomenologically as a representation within the therapist. Over time, the therapist struggles to build and maintain this representation and looks to the group members' behavior to confirm or deny this internal conception. Like the parent of an unborn child who derives meaning from every movement and sound in utero, the group therapist of the nascent group sees every patient response as a sign that the group is either progressing or dissolving (Sandel & Johnson, 1983, pp. 132-133).

Leading such a group, therefore, presents challenges quite different from facilitating groups of alert and responsive elders who develop a group identity. In groups with the confused, the entire burden is on the therapist to make the group happen, and often to make sense out of the members' fragmented expressions. The therapist may experience him/herself like an unsuspecting protagonist in a Marx brothers' movie in which nonsensical events occur randomly.

> *Therapist*: How about if we go around and remind each other of our names?
> *Lil*: Okay.
> *Therapist*: Okay. You want to start?
> *Lil*: No, you start.
> *Therapist*: Okay, my name is Susan.

Lil: My name is Ohugb one second . . . My name is Lil Wallersuell.
Therapist: You are Lillie . . .
Lil: Uh uh graceful about my brother.
Therapist: Your name is Lillie Waller.
Lil: Yes (smiles), that's right.
Therapist: Okay, your name . . .
Gerald: Hello Suzie and Lillie. My name is Gerald, Gerald Nussbaum. But don't say "bum," it's "baum." (Laughs).
Therapist: Next to Gerald we have . . . what's your name?
Morris: Mygayg.
Therapist: What's your name?
Morris: Iyodn . . .
Therapist: Morris . . . you are Morris.
Gerald: He doesn't hear well.
Therapist: Your name is Morris . . .
Gerald: Can he see?
Therapist: Your name is Morris . . .
Gerald: You Morris?
Morris: No!

In such instances, the therapist may feel frustrated at the unresponsiveness of the group to his/her efforts and the apparently random verbalizations. The simplicity of a task such as saying one's name seems to become a monumental challenge. The interminable pace of the activity created by the need to encourage each person's participation intensifies the therapist's struggle against his/her impatient desires to move on. Finally, the tremendous effort required by the therapist to achieve such apparently minor progress may leave the therapist feeling depleted, sharing the sense of impoverishment displayed by group members.

Nascent groups with the confused elderly are dependent upon external organizers, such as music, rhythm, repetitive activities, group rituals, and familiar structures in order to maintain themselves. Their success is based on the therapist's ability to utilize these organizing tools to stimulate responses and create meaningful links among the participants. In the following example, the therapist uses the familiar structure of "taking turns" to promote social awareness in the beginning of the session:

Therapist: Would anyone like to give us an exercise to get warmed up with this morning? (no response) May, do you have an exercise we can do?

May: (Silently offers an exercise.)

Therapist: (pleased) Good!

May: Stretch ourselves.

Therapist: Stretch ourselves way up . . .

May: Up and down.

Therapist & May: Up and down.

Therapist: Let's say it all together.

All: Up and down (repeating, stretching arms up and down).

George: Up to heaven and down.

All: Up and down.

Therapist: Up to heaven? Up to heaven and down.

Louise: Wow.

All: Up to heaven and down.

Therapist: (Everyone applauds the previous exercise.) Okay, could somebody give us another one? Thank you May. Could you show us another one, Jean?

May: (Mutters something indecipherable.)

Jean: I want one for her (nods towards May).

Therapist: She just gave us one.

May: (Towards Jean) She just nice and . . .

Jean: Well (to May), you already gave us one. Well, then we can't get another one from you.

Therapist: That's right. Now it's your turn.

George: She's going to fall off that chair (looking at Ethel) if she slides any further down.

Therapist: (a little impatiently) She's fine, George.

George: She's down too far.

Therapist: She's fine. You're okay, aren't you Ethel?

Ethel: I'm fine.

Therapist: Jean, it's your turn.

Jean: I'm fine.

Therapist: Can you show us an exercise?

Jean: No, I never did an exercise.

Therapist: Okay, George, can you show us one?

George: Ah, by what?

Therapist: Can you show us an exercise?

George: Everybody follow . . . up and down . . . slowly but surely . . . in the back of you . . . that's it . . . come back again and you straighten out again down, flat hands . . . up again . . . beautiful! Everybody gets a medal, the medal will be sent to them, after we get them.

Jean: (Giggles.)

May: (Smiles.)

Louise: When do each one ticawise.

George: Very good, everybody did it fine. Give them a big hand.

All: (Applaud.)

It is evident from this verbatim account that the therapist was working very hard to maintain the linking structure. Presented with a profoundly fragmented, nonsensical, and chaotic human environment, the therapist clings to the structures that provide organization to the experience, such as the applause and exercises. The slightest distraction, one person sliding down in a chair, a fleeting loose association, a word or gesture, has the potential to disrupt the group's activity. Furthermore, it is almost impossible for the therapist to predict when disruptions will occur, since many result from disorganized thoughts. The therapist's tenacious adherence to the structure is essential for even a minimal sense of coherence in such a group. Following the digression created by George's concern about Ethel, there was a feeling of relief when the group resumed its exercises, as expressed in George's comment about deserving a medal for accomplishing the stated task. Indeed, at this point the therapist also felt that she deserved a medal for persevering with the task structure in the face of potential disintegration.

FRAMING MEANINGFUL COMMUNICATION

Many institutionalized elderly who are victims of irreversible cognitive impairments remain sensitive to affective states long after they have lost the capacity for logical verbal expression. When the therapist responds to the affect being expressed in movement therapy sessions by structuring experiences in which feelings can be identified, labeled, and shared, cognitive reorganization may occur in even the most confused person. The task for the therapist is to develop the actions and interactions into a meaningful communication. Seemingly random associations that are stimulated by the movement activity may, with effort, result in a coherent communicative exchange.

CLINICAL EXAMPLE: THE ALL-TOGETHER GROUP

The following clinical example is from a special Therapeutic Group Program (T.G.P.) that was designed as an interdisciplinary effort of the staff in a nursing home. Music, movement, and simple food preparation were chosen as the major activities for the group. Each session was conducted by a pair of staff members who shared the task of leading the group and organizing the activities. Each patient was assessed for their current level of mental functioning before entering the program. Initially eight patients were selected for the group, each with a diagnosis of senile dementia, two with Alzheimer's type. The median age was 80 years old.

A small activity room with a bathroom was chosen as the ideal space for the program. A portable phonograph, foam ball, a large table for refreshments, and a coffee maker were the basic supplies used. The group met three times each week in the late afternoon, since change of shift was usually difficult for the patients. The staff quickly realized that the usual method of rounding up people individually for an activity would not work. As soon as each person arrived in the room where nothing was happening, they would wander out as the next person came in. Instead, the staff utilized a "group gather," in which they started at one end of the building and collected patients as they progressed down the hall. Because patients themselves were involved in encouraging others to attend, resistance quickly disappeared. Gathering time was reduced to ten minutes. A focus of group identity built around the fact that "We come here together, we do things together, and we leave together." The group soon was named the "All-Together Group."

After an initial warm-up period in which the participants reminded each other of their names, took turns leading exercises, and explored different kinds of sounds, the therapist began to focus on the feelings being expressed in the sounds and movements.

Therapist: How about an "O" sound?
All: OOOOHHHH!

George: Very pretty. That's very good. Give a good hand for that. (Applause)

Therapist: Can we say "oh" as if we're surprised?

All: "OH"

George: Oh no! (Everyone starts saying, "oh no.") Everybody did it, everybody did it!

Therapist: What is something that you might say "oh no" about? What might happen that would make you say, "Oh no!"

George: Oh no, don't wipe your nose! (Others echo "oh no")

Therapist: Wait a minute. Jean was about to say something. What would you say it to?

Jean: Oh no, but you nother little question at the end.

Therapist: Yes, I asked if you could think of a situation where you might say "Oh no." What kind of things might happen when you say that?

George: You're scared. Your situation.

Jean: Too much.

Therapist: You're scared? Something that's too much?

Jean: When there's something that's too much, then there's gone to . . . oooh.

Robert: Oh nooooo.

George: Too much.

Jean: Don't lose the nooo.

Robert: Nooo.

Therapist: How about for you May? When would you say, "OH NO?"

May: Oh no!

Therapist: When might you say that? What kind of thing would happen that would make you say that?

May: When you drop something that you value a good deal.

George: Very good. Very good.

Therapist: Did that ever happen to you, that you dropped something that you valued a lot?

All: (Some muttering.)

Therapist: Did that ever happen to anybody, that you dropped something like a dish or a bowl or a vase that somebody gave you, and it breaks?

Jean: Certainly. Any one can think of that.

Therapist: And then you might say, if that happened, if you drop something that you value . . .

Jean: Then you have that gone.
Therapist: And then you might say, oh no! (quietly). Oh no!
Ethel: Oh no (echoing therapist's quality).

This theme continued as each group member contributed a sentence or a non-sequitur involving the element of surprise. George then introduced the issue of disappointment.

Therapist: Did anything surprise you recently?
George: That's right. You could have a surprise or a disappointment almost anytime.
Therapist: Have you been disappointed recently?
George: Well, everybody is in life . . .
May: (Interrupting) Oh yes, surely . . .You can say that again. (The energy level and attention increases in the group.)
George: Everybody gets a disappointment through life.
Ethel: (Taps her foot.)
Therapist: Did you have any recently? What's been a recent disappointment?
George: Well, you don't have to remember, I don't remember. It's a general thing, otherwise you have to point out what it was and so on.
Therapist: May, do you have a recent disappointment that you remember?
May: Sometimes.
Therapist: Sometimes? I guess we're all disappointed sometimes.
May: Yes we are. You expect someone and you think they're going to come, and then for some reason, they aren't coming in. You're so happy at the door, you heard a knock at the door, but someone opens the door and . . .
Jean: It wasn't there!
May: Yeah, oh no!
Jean: Oh no!
May: You didn't mean to say "oh no," but it came right out!
All: Oh no! (sympathetically)

The group continued to explore movements and sounds that expressed disappointment. A familiar closing ritual was introduced in which all held hands and swayed together while making sounds; in this session the sounds were solacing "aaahs" as a response to the theme of disappointment that had prevailed.

Of clinical significance is the fact that the feeling of disappointment, although close to being concrete, was never really attached to a person or object. The therapist was obviously trying to elicit a specific situation or reason to frame the feeling of disappointment and afford it more concrete meaning. However, although all the participants were experiencing the affect, the struggle for a cognitive link was never achieved. The therapist experienced a diffuse feeling of mutuality with the group when they were all exclaiming "oh no" in unison. Differentiating and articulating individual's associations to the affect was fraught with difficulty and increased the potential for fragmentation. In addition, the therapist's attempts to lead the group into more complex modes of communication emphasized their cognitive deficits.

The challenge for the therapist in such a group is to mediate the cognitive demands with a periodic return to sensorimotor unison activities that form the secure base for trust and linking. If participants experience the activity as too frustrating or demanding, they may try to leave or retreat into self-soothing behaviors. Thus the therapist must continually return to simple, familiar movements and sounds, and must not focus on any one individual for too long.

When the Therapeutic Group Program began, the participants were only able to do very simple movement activities such as clapping their hands and imitating the leader's motions. Refreshments were limited to coffee and cookies. As people became more familiar with the group, they began to take initiative in tasks such as leading movements, throwing the ball to each other, and serving refreshments. The staff introduced (with suggestions from the patients) food activities such as slicing fruit, icing cupcakes, spreading jam on crackers. There was some improvement over time in their ability to perform these tasks in an organized way. For example, the first time icing cupcakes was attempted, several people ate the icing and the cupcake separately. Several months later, everyone followed the instruction to ice the cupcake before eating it.

Patient's social interactions outside of the group measurably improved. Prior to the implementation of the program, several people were unable to tolerate large social events. After the program had been meeting for four months, the patients were able to attend these social occasions when the staff provided support by gathering them together, saying, "We are all going to a party together."

Although the Therapeutic Group Program does not offer a cure for confusion and disorientation, such a program provides a caring, structured environment in which people can organize their day and their social interactions. The relationships that develop, even when people do not remember each other's names, do enrich the quality of people's lives in the nursing home. Initially, the staff thought that refreshments would be a major motivation for people to attend the group. One day the therapist told one woman that they were going to have fresh strawberries as part of their activity. She replied, "I'm not coming to the group to eat strawberries; I'm coming to be with you!"

THERAPEUTIC IMPLICATIONS

An area of concern for the therapist is coping with the feelings of loneliness and hopelessness that are evoked by this work. The long-term care field stresses the importance of developing programs for mentally impaired residents of nursing homes. Stability and predictability of activities and staff are increasingly recognized as essential factors in program design (Berger, 1985; AAHA, 1985). How do these caregivers sustain their energy and motivation in the daily encounter with the confused aged? An understanding of the modalities that are most successful in reaching confused clients, an effort towards teamwork, sensitivity to affective states, and an appreciation of small behavioral changes all contribute to the caregiver's ability to sustain motivation and achieve therapeutic goals. The following are suggestions and implications for designing therapeutic group programs with the cognitively impaired elderly.

1. *Choose appropriate modalities.* Tasks that are complex or require a high level of cognitive organization are inappropriate for groups with confused people. Activities that provide simplicity, repetition, and sensory stimulation are ideal: therefore, music and movement are the choice therapeutic modalities for the confused aged. Dancing, making music, and reminiscing stimulate cognitive reorganization in the confused person and often reveal vestiges of their "personhood," which, in turn, evokes hopeful and warm feelings in the therapist. In order to be helpful to a client, the therapist must experience hope, and must derive some gratification from the work.

It is essential that the therapist become as open as possible, within himself, to the experiencing of whatever gratifications this work, which initially tends to be so deprivational, so engendering of feelings of futility and discouragement, can come to afford him . . . The therapist's becoming aware of these gratifications comes to engender hope in both participants that the therapy will prove meaningful'' (Searles, 1977, p. 502).

Through the medium of movement, the dance therapist often discovers aspects of the person that may not initially be apparent to ward staff during routine care. A creative spark or spontaneous expression may emerge in a movement session that affirms the patient's humanity. It is essential for all staff to be made aware of such responses so that all "humanizing" information is available in developing team treatment plans.

2. *Use a team approach.* The ability of even the most dedicated and motivated caregiver to withstand solitary forays into the world of the confused is limited, at best. The therapist may alternately experience feelings of intense closeness to and alienation from group members. Unison movement and sound tends to promote feelings of mutuality and cohesion, while attempts at more differentiated conversation or activity will intensify the members' struggle for relatedness. It is unrealistic to expect one therapist to continually work alone with groups of the mentally impaired elderly, even in movement and music. A team approach that provides mutual support and the opportunity for communicating with another rational person is essential for staff well-being. Having another person with whom the primary therapist can maintain eye contact and nonverbal communication is helpful for survival, particularly in chaotic or disturbing sessions.

3. *Be aware of affective communication.* Because the cognitively impaired elderly often retain their sensitivity to affective expression despite their deterioration in cognition, the development of therapeutic relationships depend upon nonverbal cues. Touch, facial expression, and especially tone of voice are more critical to communication than the verbal content. Saying "How are you?" will communicate the meaning that you care when it is said in a soft tone of voice with a friendly smile, even though the patient has not understood the words. Yet this does not mean that one should assume the confused person can not understand verbal communication at all. By assuming that everyone understands in their own way, the therapist contributes to the atmosphere of safety, acceptance, and respect. Since confused people are sensitive to humiliation and are likely to misinterpret verbal directives, staff should not talk *about* people as

if they are not present or do not understand. One woman who had been excluded from many activities by residents and staff due to her severe confusion remarked in a clearer moment, "I only want to be with people who want to be with me!"

4. *Abandon traditional notions of cure.* When working with the elderly who are victims of irreversible dementia, one must abandon traditional notions of cure. Goals should be consistent with the patient's functional assessment and prognosis. Providing a consistent environment, stimulating reminiscing, and maintaining social contacts are important elements of any psychosocial treatment plan. Periods of cognitive reorganization and improved social functioning may occur during structured groups; however, the therapist in his/her enthusiasm must be wary not to convey misleading messages to family members who are all too ready to hear "cure." As previously mentioned, the therapeutic task is to create a life-sustaining and enlivening environment in which maximum functioning is supported.

CONCLUSION

Understanding the distinct process and organization of the nascent group may be useful in diminishing negative attitudes about groups with geriatric patients. Judging the effectiveness of these groups by standards that are usually applied to activities and creative arts therapy is inappropriate, and leads to a devaluation of group members, of the therapy, and of the therapist.

These people, given the severity of their cognitive deficits, require a structured environment that is based on sensorimotor experiences in order to give temporary coherence to their feelings and to their relationships. In these groups, people do respond with improved behavior under the guidance of a skilled, caring leader. However, this improved social and behavioral functioning may not generalize to other situations in institutional life where similar support is not present. However, the dependence on special groups and environments does not mitigate their importance in the lives of the cognitively impaired elderly, but rather points out the necessity for providing them in therapeutic settings. The therapeutic group session becomes an island of relative calm and sanity in a day otherwise beset by confusion and anxiety, providing momentary reassurance and supporting the person's courage to go on. What more profound service can a therapy offer?

III. The Arts and Communitas

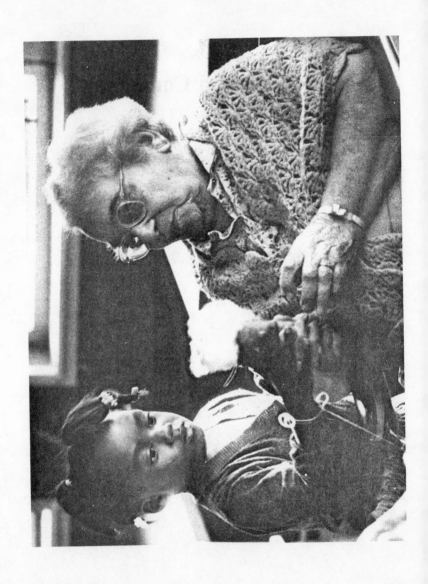

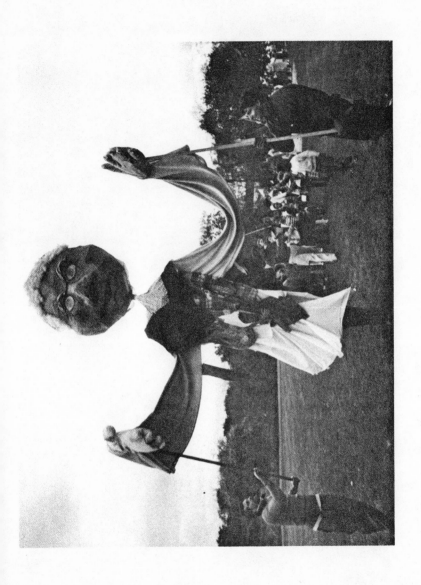

Chapter Ten
Creating and Playing: Bridges for Intergenerational Communication

Susan L. Sandel

The positive effects of bringing old and young together in intergenerational programs have been highly lauded, and many such programs have received a great deal of media attention. With support from advocacy groups, as well as public and private foundations, intergenerational events are occurring across the country. Testimonials from people of all ages provide compelling evidence of the benefits to those who are involved in such programs. However, the task of structuring intergenerational programs with widely disparate groups of children and the elderly for the purposes of encouraging learning and the development of meaningful relationships is indeed a challenge. For example, a group of elders in a senior center and a class of gifted junior-high-school students require different modes of communication than do preschoolers interacting with nursing-home residents.

In our intergenerational program, Project TOUCH, which began as an exchange between the New Haven Convalescent Center and the neighboring Barnard School, we ventured to bring together the residents of a long-term care residential geriatric facility and students from an inner-city elementary school. The proximity of the school to the convalescent center (literally in its backyard) provided an irresistible challenge to develop an ongoing, interactive neighborhood program.

The "touch" in Project TOUCH stands for a specific set of goals:

Originally published in *Design for Arts in Education* (1984), September-October, No. 86, 32-35. Reprinted by permission of the Helen Dwight Reid Educational Foundation. Published by Heldref Publications, 4000 Albermarle Street, N.W., Washington, D.C., 20016. Copyright © 1984.

Teaching each other new skills through shared experiences

Opening our doors to promote intergenerational communication

Understanding our differences and what we can offer each other

Community-building in our own neighborhood through involvement

Helping one another feel better about ourselves

The residents of the New Haven Convalescent Center, who range in age from 70 to 101, are predominately white, middle class with a diversity of ethnic and religious affiliations. The conditions that precede their placement in the nursing home range from age-specific ailments (seriously impaired vision, hearing, organic brain disease, inability to thrive independently) to Alzheimer's disease, coronary disease, stroke, cancer, multiple sclerosis, Parkinson's disease, diabetes, and psychological problems related to aging. All people who live and work in this kind of setting are continuously confronted with issues concerning helplessness, dependency, and death.

The children who attend the Barnard School are predominately inner-city, poor to lower-middle class, black and Hispanic, and are in grades kindergarten through five. Their academic and social maturation, with a few exceptions, are below grade level. Many are latch-key children in single parent families with a mother or grandmother as the head-of-household. We discovered that since the age of the parent(s) and grandparent(s) is often quite young, many of them have had no contact with an old person (i.e., 70 years or older).

How were we to build bridges for communication between these isolated communities-within-a-community that had no previous contact? What did these two disparate populations have in common?

Both these groups of elders and children have either impaired or poorly developed verbal skills, and both suffer from low self-esteem. Many of the nursing-home residents experience a feeling of shame in relation to the limitations incurred by their various handicaps. A majority of the children, who live in environments that do not support academic achievement, view themselves as incapable of learning. It was evident that arts experiences that did not rely primarily on highly developed verbal skills, such as movement, music, mime, and visual arts, would be the most likely modes of interaction for these two groups. We realized that it was important for the participants to build a repertoire of shared experiences from which relationships could develop.

THE MODEL

Project TOUCH, which is now entering its fourth year, is based on an arts workshop model. That is, trained creative arts therapists and educators conduct time-limited workshops (6-14 weeks) in a specific arts modality for a preselected group of children and adults. All sessions are scheduled in consultation with the participating teachers, taking into consideration curriculum content, the school calendar, and the convalescent center yearly calendar. In addition to the ongoing workshops, there are also monthly large-group programs (50 children and adults) and an annual community ritual involving the entire school, nursing home, and contributing artists and arts therapists. Most workshops are held at the New Haven Convalescent Center, but residents also go to the school to participate in assemblies and give musical performances by their own singing group.

Following is a brief description of the unique contribution of each of the arts modalities to the program.

RHYTHMIC MOVEMENT:
THE FIRST MODE OF COMMUNICATION

Rhythm is the fundamental element which facilitates communication through body movement and fosters social unity. The rhythm of dance was used early in the history of mankind to bridge isolation and achieve a sense of community (Bartenieff, 1972). Rhythmic movement has been an effective mode for fostering learning experiences with young children and communication among nursing home residents (Rowen, 1963).

Project TOUCH began with a group of the elderly and a class of kindergartners participating in movement activities together. These groups were led by trained dance-movement therapists and movement educators who facilitated activities that encouraged interaction. Mutually-recognizable actions such as throwing a ball, shaking hands, jumping rope, and throwing a kiss were incorporated into rhythmic games. At first, the children tended to look for peers when movements involving touch were introduced. As they became more familiar with the participants and the activities, they began to shake hands with the elderly and eventually, to hug and kiss them. By the end of the initial eight-week period, there was spontaneous hugging, kissing, and conversing between the adults and children. Dance-movement has continued to be the basic mode of interaction with children in the lower grades and the older people.

CREATING A SHARED REPERTOIRE THROUGH SONG

Singing together has been one of the most important arts activities in our community-building. Each class that has participated in on-going music workshops with the nursing-home residents has developed its own music rituals. "Hello" songs, "goodbye" songs, "naming" songs, "travelling" songs—a varied repertoire, but one which is shared and remembered by the participants long after the workshop is over. This has made it possible for a third-grader to come back when in fourth grade and have a shared knowledge base with some of the elderly upon which to renew their relationships.

When an "intergenerational gate" was installed in the fence that adjoins the two institutions in 1983, a "gate" song was composed and taught to everyone. During our 1984 community event, all 250 children and most of the older people who had participated the year before, sang the gate song with enthusiasm and delight. The songs have thus begun to establish a continuity to the program and form the basis of shared rituals.

EXPLORING CAPABILITIES IN CLAY

A third-grade class was selected to fashion a clay mural with a group of elders built on the theme "Our Neighborhood." Both the children and the elderly enjoyed the preparation of the material; the pounding, or "wedging" of the clay, was a wonderful opportunity for expressing aggression by young and old alike. Both populations, however, were hesitant to create a product. Fears of failure and incompetence in using their hands were shared by the majority of the young and old. The art therapist created a non-judgmental, open environment in which each individual was free to express his or her

images of the neighborhood. The secondary title of the group was
" I Am Loveable and Capable," which the therapist continually
reinforced through discussion and blackboard displays. The classroom teacher took this theme back to school, where the children
wrote mini-essays on this topic. Ultimately, they did produce a clay
collage expressing a wide range of individual creativity. The process resulted in the old and young helping each other to not only
complete the task, but also to validate feelings of self-worth and
competency.

COMMUNICATION THROUGH DRAMATIC PLAY

Storytelling, puppetry, and mime have been the vehicles for intergenerational dramatic play about issues that were diffcult for both
the young and old to articulate. For example, a story told by a drama
therapist and acted out through sound effects and movement
concerning a Thanksgiving turkey looking for a family's table
touched upon, in a playful manner, both the children's and elderly's
anxiety about impending holidays. The search by a little girl puppet
for a grandmother puppet that was disguised as a witch elicited
responses about how an ugly or scary appearance may be deceptive
and may mask a beautiful person. The children subsequently each
paired up with a "grandparent" in the room, producing smiles,
hugs, and lively conversation. Because dramatic play permits the
participants to distance themselves from painful or difficult topics
through role-playing and make-believe, it provides a helpful
creative medium for dealing with previously unarticulated issues
(Johnson, 1982b).

COMMUNITY BUILDING THROUGH THEATRICAL EVENTS

A major annual theatrical event and other mini-events and festivals
have served to concretize the values of intergenerational community
building and sharing. David Cole conceptualizes theatre as "an opportunity to experience imaginative life as physical presence."
(Cole, 1975). In attempting to use the arts to foster interaction
among verbally-limited people, the manifestation of ideals, values,
and goals in the form of theatre has communicative impact. Par-

ticipatory theatrical events such as pageants, parades, balloon flys, and giant puppet plays serve as bonding experiences to the imagined idea of the sense of community for which we are striving. The installation of the intergenerational gate in the fence which separated the school from the nursing home is a concrete, yet also symbolic, representation of the link that has been established. It also provides a vehicle for the organization of observable rituals.

GROUP LEADERS: TEACHERS OR THERAPISTS?

Currently there is no specialized training program for conducting an arts workshop with six-year-olds and ninety-year-olds. It has been exceptionally challenging to the creative arts therapists and teachers who have ventured to take on the task. A combination of qualities that characterize the therapist, teacher, and artist are most ideal to meet the demands of this situation. In our experience, a cooperative team approach has been most successful. In such groups, the creative arts therapist or art teacher is the primary leader, with a classroom teacher and activities staff member as facilitators. The facilitators, who know the individuals intimately, can intervene when appropriate to help a child or older person participate. The primary leader must not only be extremely skilled in the arts medium but must be able to provide a structured, safe environment within which multiple lines of communication can develop. Although we have no formula to offer, the smoothest running groups to date have been conducted by individuals who have experience teaching both children and the elderly, have a working knowledge of group process, a broad repertoire of creative activities at their fingertips, and the ability to be spontaneous while maintaining a reliable group structure.

BENEFITS OF THE PROGRAM

There are many benefits for both the children and the older people in a program such as Project TOUCH. The children inject energy and life into the nursing home each time they cross the threshold. Some residents feel that the program is a highlight of the facility itself and contributes to an overall atmosphere of liveliness. Especially the more alert residents of the New Haven Convalescent Center recognize that *they* are contributing to the quality of the lives and education of the children. Since the program's inception, several former public school teachers who reside at the center have become involved not only with the children but also in advising and counseling the teachers.

In addition to the social experience of being with people of different backgrounds and generations, the program directly impacts on the children's academic learning. The teachers incorporate the contents of the arts workshops into their classroom curriculum through the use of experience charts, discussion, drawing, and writing exercises. Often compositions are sent back to the nursing home and posted on bulletin boards where the children can read them when they return. One teacher told us that she was sure she had the only fourth-grade class in New Haven in which every child can spell "convalescent." The arts workshops offer the children an alternative mode of learning which the teachers, principal, and program coordinator believe can significantly contribute to their educational development. Although the younger grades have a music class as part of their school day, other arts classes have been eliminated due to budgetary constraints. Therefore, Project TOUCH offers curriculum enrichment to children who might not otherwise have the exposure to the arts in their elementary school years.

The meaning of Project TOUCH for the children seems to vary widely with their individual age, intelligence, sensitivity, and curiosity. For some, it means a chance to escape from the confines of the classroom and have fun. For others, the reward is the satisfying feeling of brightening the lives of the institutionalized elderly. For yet others, Project TOUCH provides experiences which boost self-esteem and opens new vistas for learning.

Chapter Eleven
Intergenerational Movement Therapy: A Leadership Challenge

Betsy Mason-Luckey
Susan L. Sandel

This chapter will focus on the twelve sessions of music and movement which comprised one part of Project TOUCH. Approximately
twelve kindergarten children and eighteen residents met weekly for
forty-five minutes with a dance-movement therapist and the classroom teacher. Structured movement activities, folk songs and games
were the major vehicles for expression and interaction.

Because both elders and children have impaired or poorly developed verbal skills, dance-movement was chosen as the basic mode
of interaction for this intergenerational program. Rhythmic games
and folk songs offered a potential basis for developing a shared
repertoire of experiences from which relationships could develop.

STRUCTURE OF THE SESSIONS

The therapist's goal is to create a safe and caring environment
with activities that engage both the young and old. The experiences
have to be meaningful for both groups while encouraging spontaneous interaction. Movement and music can not be too complex,
but also not so simple that the children or adults become bored. It is
important for all participants to experience a feeling of accomplishment and enrichment.

The challenge is to harmonize the bouncy and erratic energies of
the children with the lower energies of the residents and to allow
space for youthful expansiveness without overwhelming their aged
counterparts. It is necessary to create a structure which appreciates

Originally published in *The Arts in Psychotherapy* (1985), Vol. 12, No. 4, 257-262.
Reprinted by permission of ANKHO International, Inc.

the bound and limited movement qualities of the elderly, yet does not inhibit the quick, here-and-now responsiveness of the children.

Structure, simplicity and repetition are key variables in planning intergenerational movement sessions. The circle formation creates the first sense of a container and structure for the group. Children are made aware of their limits by alternating young and old within the boundary of chairs and wheelchairs. The circle allows the children to maximize their movement space while keeping the adults in view and accessible to all. The leader is seen by all and the leadership can easily be passed around.

Simple rituals define the beginning, middle and end of each session. A greeting which involves the whole group in rhythmical song and movement awakens all to the presence of each other in the group. Repetition of certain songs and games from week to week is extremely important to lend continuity to the program and support the group's identity. For example, a favorite greeting ritual is "Funga Alafia, Ashay, Ashay," an African welcoming chant (learned from Susan Cambique) in which the same words are repeated over and over while gestures vary and alter the meaning of each verse. Folk songs and singing games are ideally suited for an intergenerational group of this kind since they teach skills and activate the reflective process. They quickly engage young and old because they are lively and simple. Often the melody is comprised of only two to five notes; frequently they are in the pentatonic scale which is indigenous to almost every culture.

Simple games requiring modest skills can be developed to encourage learning names and touching each other. The children may temporarily become the primary movers while the adults reflect or respond to their moves. Skipping around the inside of the circle to music and stopping in front of a new partner encourages new relationships. Simple movement exercises such as mirroring, touching toes or fingertips, bowing, nodding and stretching with a partner acquaint the participants in structured and playful ways. Lively and rhythmical music engages the older participants while satisfying the child's need to be energetic.

The farewell and departure of the children is a difficult transition for all. In each session, small separations occur within the activities, but the actual parting for the week can evoke feelings of sadness. An orderly, ritualistic quality to the departure helps contain the feelings and activities of disengaging. Moving together to music enhances the experience of unity prior to the separation. Farewells can be punctuated by a march or other familiar activity and can recapitulate the opening ritual, but with the goal of saying goodbye to each person.

MOVEMENT THEMES AND ACTIVITIES

When participants are warmed up and reacquainted through familiar rituals, they are ready to focus on a topic of mutual interest. The next task is to generate a theme which is engaging to both populations. Ideally, the theme emerges from the group as they express their feelings and associations to the activity they have just experienced. Life experiences that people of all ages have in common, such as seasons, birth, growth, nature, provide the opportunity for the adults to reminisce and teach and for the children to demonstrate and learn.

> For example, one windy March day the topic was, not surprisingly, the wind. A forest of trees was created inside the circle by several children shaping their bodies in appropriate configurations. These 'trees' bent and twisted against the imaginary force of the winds, enacted by residents and children in the circle who made wind sounds and movements with their arms. We also put scarves on the trees which waved in the winds like 'leaves' and then subsided as the winds died down. One resident became a tree in her wheelchair and everyone clapped for her.

As previously mentioned, since the participants' capacity for verbally sharing and processing their experience is limited, responses may lead quickly into another action, such as in the following example.

> A discussion about letting go of winter, with its positive and negative aspects, prompted a resident to burst into song: "Gonna Lay My Burden Down, Down By The Riverside." Young and old revealed the burdens they would let go—boots, colds, cold weather, which we acted out through gesture and mime.

Feelings

In another session, the theme of feelings led to a discussion about how people comfort themselves and others. The therapist facilitated this theme by introducing her own childhood Teddy Bear. The idea of the Teddy Bear as a friend emerged and, little by little, several children told of their favorite soft toy or special place or blanket. Some of the residents just listened, but several could recall a favorite toy from their own childhoods quite clearly, thus giving glimpses of events and characteristics of their earlier lives and respecting the spirit of this kind of affectionate and imaginal play.

An obvious singing game to evolve out of this topic is the jumping-rope chant, "Teddy Bear, Teddy Bear," (Fowke, 1969, p. 49).

The movement therapist described this activity as follows:

> While the children acted out the words in the center of the circle, the residents joined in the singing and clapped to the rhythm or enacted the words as best they could in their seats. We also worked in partners, young with old, and sped up the tempo. We then tried it in slow motion and in larger motions. In the end, I passed my old Teddy Bear around the circle to reaffirm symbolically that we all have a friend inside, if not outside, and that, although one may become old and raggedy in appearance, we are still loved despite the markings of age and experience.

Illness

An obvious concern for such an intergenerational group is illness. Absenteeism among both young and old stimulates anxieties about illness and death. As interesting as ailments might be for both populations, perhaps more engaging are the remedies. Old and young alike can share what mother or grandmother or nurse does when he or she has the flu, the whooping cough or a cold.

"John Brown's Baby" (Nelson, 1977, p. 24) is a useful song for this topic as it can be sung and acted out easily, and can support any amount of improvisation. In a way the song becomes a ritualization and celebration of the healing process. The group all actively share a personal illness (such as coughing with the whooping cough), and then communally share in the healing process ("his mother gave him sweet cough medicine"), no matter how unusual it might be.

The melody to the song is well-known to young and old: the chorus to the "Battle Hymn of the Republic."

Birthdays

Birthdays are as great a cause of celebration and community at the convalescent center as they are for young school children. After one reaches a certain age, there is often tremendous pride in each advancing year. Each month brings a party day for all residents having their birthday during that month. The whole community comes together; names are read and often ages are revealed. There is an enormous cake, punch, lots of singing of old and familiar songs. Any child is thrilled by such a birthday.

The topic of birthdays facilitates the celebration of diversity in ages. New ties can be made when birthday months and days are revealed. Children love to remember their own birth date and to know who shares the same month or day.

A birthday rhyme challenges everyone's memory and requires some skill in the enactment. One person is chosen to walk around the inside of the circle touching eight people consecutively on the beat while everyone else chants the words. (Fowke, 1969, p. 55.)

The eighth person has the opportunity to tell his or her birthday to the group. If the eighth person is a child, the children change places and number eight, the birthday person, now becomes the "counter." If the eighth person is a resident, then the child on his or her right is chosen to be the next counter. If this person is a child or resident who is shy or unable to speak, then the group acts supportively by acknowledging the person's presence and perhaps telling the birthday.

Fantasy and Hope

A singing game which engages an intergenerational group is "Bluebird Through My Window" (Fowke & Seeger, 1948, pp. 24, 118-119). This song appeals to the spirit of young and old alike, creating a bond between the generations through a fanciful dream image in which all may participate. The tune is very simple, the idea is cyclical, and the story repeats itself over and over.

Traditionally, everyone stands in a circle holding hands. The windows through which the Bluebird must "fly" are the spaces between each person, framed by the bridges of their connected arms.

The person who is the "Bluebird" flies (walks, skips, runs) in and out through each window consecutively all around the circle. As the song ends, the "bird" lands and changes places with the nearest window-maker and the cycle begins again.

The configuration may be adapted to suit the needs of people in chairs and wheelchairs by making smaller inner circles of four or five individuals. Standing children hold hands with the residents, creating a network of windows that encourage focus and collaboration. Participants experience delight at having the "blue bird" come through their window and in getting the opportunity to be the "Blue bird."

TIME: FINDING A COMMON RHYTHM

Kindergarteners and elders have different relationships to the elements of time and life's rhythm. A common rhythm of the very old and infirm resident of the convalescent center is that of the pause, or waiting. When one is not ambulatory, one is more dependent on the timing and mercy of others to have one's needs met. This sense of waiting, patient waiting, is one which these people especially know and live. Waiting to be aroused in the morning, waiting for breakfast, waiting to be dressed; then, waiting for lunch, for companionship, waiting to be taken to the bathroom, waiting for solitude, waiting for attention and waiting for sleep. One begins to accept a state of passivity in relation to the environment. One is more a passenger of the moment and the movement, no longer the carrier of it, as is the child. Furthermore, the past and what it held has at least as much importance as the present.

The common rhythm of children, especially an active five-year-old, is activity of almost any kind, reflecting all the youthful energy and feeling of the moment. Even sitting still is active. Within the framework of adult time, the rhythms of children form, develop and change at a rapid pace. They own every moment and yesterday, today and tomorrow are nearly indistinguishable. Children's sensitivities are exposed, and their bodies reflect all that creates the present moment.

Both the child and the resident of a convalescent center need certain expectations to be met in order to maintain a sense of balance and security in the flow of time. Ritual and repetition provide a necessary container for the dichotomous relationship of the old and young to time.

Singing games provide room for individual patterns and playfulness. Within the framework of a musical game, the child may have to wait while the older person takes his or her turn. It is safe to switch roles. The child, through this experience, gains new controls and a new perspective on the order and timing of actions. The older person, in the safety of a sequence and a structure, is drawn into the action and potential control of the present.

By keeping the beginning and ending of the session very structured and simple, the middle part of the session can develop with a lot of flexibility. Knowing and understanding that there is a ritual for departure helps everyone to make the transition to real time and their own rhythms.

GUIDELINES FOR LEADERS

Some guidelines for conserving and guiding the disparate energies in an intergenerational group are: limitation, focus, simplification and repetition.

Boundaries are automatically set by the circle of chairs and wheelchairs and by the small amount of time in which there is to work. While there is some space in the middle for the energies and the expansiveness of the children's movement, there is adequate space on the perimeter for the old to move freely. Directions from the leader limit how many children can move in the center at once or how they can circle the inside of the ring. There is a surprising amount of movement and inventiveness that can arise from these limitations.

Often the minds of young children take them on fast journeys which one must ride out or share with them; they taste quickly and move on, in contrast to the older person's desire for focus and savoring the moment which carries so much of the past. In an intergenerational movement group, focusing on a theme, a game or a topic helps the young to stay with a subject and the old to get involved, even catch up. Encouraging a direction brings the fruits of the child's imagination and activity together with the depth and reflective contribution of the aging person.

The physical limitations that five-year-olds must exert or experience with peers is quite different than the controls they must master when touching or moving with the resident of a nursing home. Here simple directions, simple formats for moving together, such as mirroring or partnering, help the children to channel their energies. Too much, too fast, tends to confuse both the children and the adults.

Music is a great catalyst in bringing the two energy extremes together. Rhythmic movement, repetition and patterning encourage the development of focus and skills and bring everyone closer in time and energy.

THERAPIST'S ROLE

The management functions of the dance-movement therapist in an intergenerational group are particularly challenging. The therapist must mediate the range of simplicity-complexity in the group's tasks and the disparity in rhythms and energy. In contrast to the child, the residents of a nursing home are usually contending with mental and physical rigidities and disabilites. As they are carriers of personal and collective traditions, rigid patterns of movement and thought often make them resistant to change and to the sense of ''now'' which the child embraces. The confinement of a chair or wheelchair limits the kinesphere of the very old person even more. The movement therapist serves as a catalyst in extending their movements within a very limited space. Small gestures and movements are signals of full expressions of feeling and inspiration (Sandel & Johnson, 1983).

A further challenge for the therapist is to mediate his/her own role relationships to the different generations. The therapist, in the middle span of age between the very young and the very old, is the recipient of different perceptions of elders and children. The therapist may be seen simultaneously as teacher, mother, helper, and a young thing, girl, daughter. The senior author describes her experience as follows:

> The leader is in a season of his or her own; both the mother and the daughter, and teacher and student as well. I felt myself to be hostess to the children and the workshop itself, but also to have a sense of being hosted by the residents. I felt myself residing in energy level somewhere between the activity and sense of immediacy of the child and the reflective bound qualities of the much older person. I could not know or instruct them in all that went on. While I was the leader in charge, I was still a young whippersnapper.

Therapists in groups with the elderly typically experience themselves as both parent and child (Meerloo, 1955). This phenomenon is further complicated in an intergenerational group by the presence of the young children for whom the movement therapist is clearly leader, teacher and parental figure. In movement or drama groups with the elderly, the therapist often becomes the focus of the participants' efforts to re-live the past. In an intergenerational group, the past may be re-experienced through activities with the children for which the leader is a catalyst and guide. For example, in the "Bluebird" game described above, in which all the children had a chance to be a "bluebird," two residents demanded their turn:

> Charlie, who insisted upon having his turn, was pushed through all the windows in his wheelchair by two very proud youngsters. Lucy, who was ambulatory, but generally did not initiate much, decided one day that she would be the bird, to everyone's delight. She was clearly pleased with her accomplishment when she was finished and told the group, "If I was silly, then so much the better!"

A leadership style which is characterized by strong support of the rhythmic structure, a close monitoring of group interaction and the therapist's use of his/her own body action as an organizing focus is most effective in this kind of intergenerational group (Johnson, Sandel & Eicher, 1983). By being actively present with voice and body—by being willing to sing, demonstrate a movement and dare to be a little silly—the leader can encourage others to join in and share themselves in a similar way. The creation of a protective social environment with reliance on simple structures makes it possible for young and old to participate comfortably at the level of their own ability.

CONCLUSION

Bringing children into a nursing home for movement activities with the elderly, as in Project TOUCH, can be a positive experience for both groups if carefully managed. The purpose is not to challenge the aging process, but to accept it and integrate it into the children's experience. In this culture, with its emphasis on youth, extroversion and productivity, Project TOUCH offers a situation in which the contrasting values of age, introversion, patience and process can be recognized and appreciated. Furthermore, the values of play and fantasy are reinforced during these gatherings.

True sharing does not have to be forced for there is a natural attraction between young and old, actors and reflectors. The structures of music and movement games facilitate constructive relationships, vocalization, imagining, remembering and sharing. These kinds of experiences carry the whole group into a shared realm of its own creation, such as in a ritual or dream.

The children make an important contribution to the lives of the nursing home residents. The presence of these young minds and bodies revitalizes the bones and muscles and awakens the minds of the older people as they move and play together. The presence of the older people can provide an important grounding for the children's activity. In order to accommodate to an elder the child must sometimes scale down his or her energy. The child's self-control is thereby reinforced by the interest of the older person. Many children love to show off or demonstrate their abilities and to be praised by adults. Assuming a helping role in relationship to the disabled older person also supports the child's developing self-esteem and brings positive feedback for constructive behavior.

Through common musical rhythms, chanting and circle games, young and old can be present in the same "now," despite their usually different sense of the present. Children learn to understand, accept and give to their friends while the old have the chance to touch and be touched, to share themselves, to reflect and to pass on their knowledge.

Chapter Twelve
Therapeutic Rituals in the Nursing Home

David Read Johnson

Timelessness pervades the atmosphere of the nursing home at every turn. The sense of purpose, having goals toward which one strives, the experience of *becoming* rather than *having been* is challenged by the realities of retirement, isolation, and physical infirmity present among nursing home residents. Each day begins and progresses like most others. What fills the day are the basic tasks of waking, dressing, eating, elimination, and preparing for sleep. Beyond this are the daily activities and events scheduled and unscheduled, expected and unexpected, the routine and the special. The survival of the self is dependent upon to what degree these activities are experienced as personal, meaningful, and authentic, and to what extent they are gratifying and enriching, rather than depleting and rote. Otherwise the Past remains the only reservoir of self, of meaning; and turning inward the only method of achieving peace.

Yet the Present potentially has much to offer. Spontaneous conversation and visits from friends and relatives are extremely important. Scheduled groups and programs, which are discussed in other chapters of this book, also make a major contribution. Communal rituals are a third kind of activity that serve an important function in the nursing home. Rituals mediate the present and the past, the public social world and private reverie. By representing both striving and acceptance, the ritual may provide the older person with an opportunity for continued personal integration and meaningfulness. In their absence, the person's need for structure and integration often leads to the development of more and more idiosyncratic, personal rituals, such as hoarding or repetitive actions. They become increasingly self-referential and less linked to a social function. The provision of socially approved rituals allows many nursing home residents to remain linked to the world. For example, one man in a

nursing home spent all day in his room, in pajamas, obsessively col-
lecting newspapers and ruminating until he became interested in the
routine care of the new rabbit and dog introduced to the home. He is
now dressed, out of his room, talkative, and obsessively in charge of
feeding and cleaning the two animals. His need for a structuring
ritual remains; the deterioration in his social functioning has been
reversed.

In this chapter, the functions of rituals and the nature and types of
therapeutic ritual will be described. Then, a case example of a therapeutic ritual designed in a nursing home will be presented and
discussed.

FUNCTIONS OF RITUAL IN THE NURSING HOME

Typical rituals include monthly birthday celebrations, holiday
parties (e.g., Christmas, Halloween, Valentine's Day), summer
picnics, and religious ceremonies. These rituals serve many important functions.

First, rituals express and contain important human experiences
such as death, birth, achievement, and celebration. They mark off
time to allow for an orderly recognition of the passing of life. This
allows for reminiscence, encapsulation and comparison of experience from month to month or year to year. Rituals create a special place and time in which one's life can be given fresh perspective, and fundamental values and meaning can be recaptured.

Second, rituals serve as an opportunity for members of a group to
reenact their bonding to the shared social enterprise, to recreate the
group, and to reenact the pledge to the group. During rituals, each
person is asked to reaffirm their link and loyalty to the group. This
is often done through pledges spoken in unison, communal eating,
or tokens such as pins or flowers that are worn by each group
member.

Third, the establishment of a ritual over many years functions as a
reassurance that the group, through this ritual, will continue through
time beyond the death of the individual; thus, by participation in the
ritual, one transcends death.

Rituals stand in contrast to other events such as ceremonies in that
they have a predictable structure and consistency of form, they are
repeated at regular intervals, and they are sustained by a shared interest of all the community's members. Within each ritual there is
usually room for some unique contribution from certain individuals
acting as representatives of the group, such as the sermon within the

mass. However, the format of rituals is *proscribed*, either by sacred texts or tradition. It is not based on spontaneous agreement among group members. Not following the ritual correctly creates anxiety among members, who often fear it as a sign of bad luck. The "something bad" that will happen if the ritual is not followed is of course the outbreak of the disturbing emotions that the ritual has been designed to circumvent. Rituals are thus characterized by tremendous resistance to change, with members often expressing outright fear, anger, or confusion if some change is proposed.

Rituals therefore develop around issues that may threaten communal survival, and which, if uncontained, will be disturbing to its members. For example, the ritual of communion in the Catholic Church, in which members of the group reenact the murder and sacrifice of Christ by each consuming his blood and body, thereby accepting him as their savior, explicitly represents the threat to survival. The disturbing aspect of such blood sacrifice is transformed by the high moral ideals and setting of the church. Marriage ceremonies are highly ritualized due to the potential threat that the pair may have a stronger bond to each other than to the community. The ceremony must represent both the love of the couple and the control by the community. Thus, the practice in which the father gives the bride to the groom, who places his ring on her, suggests a business transaction in which property is transferred from one man to another. Modern couples who experience this imagery as disturbing often attempt to alter the ceremony to more accurately match their feelings about marriage.

Rituals vary in the degree to which they allow expression of underlying concerns and anxieties of the community. In some rituals, the disturbing element has been highly transformed so that it is barely discernible. In others, it is more accessible. Rituals involving sports, or symbols such as flags or parades, tend to be less transparent in comparison to rituals that utilize the arts such as music, art, or drama. The arts are representational forms of expression, not merely symbols that are representative of another state. The arts represent the internal life, the murky, ambiguous, constantly shifting internal world of dream, emotion, and doubt. In this way, they are transcendant, since they speak of the imaginative world. If the anxiety-provoking imagery is not sufficiently altered, then what could be moving will become disturbing.

The capacity of most nursing homes to tolerate the expression of disturbing emotions is low, so rituals are utilized to help suppress anxiety. It is not surprising that in many nursing homes, rituals remain attached only to the distant culture, often are performed in rote ways, and are avoided if they express disturbing feelings too directly. This leads to the absence of important rituals.

For example, in one Veterans Administration nursing home, the rituals that had developed over many years included Christmas, Halloween, Valentine's Day, and a summer picnic. Despite the fact that all the residents were veterans, no celebration or ritual had been planned for Veteran's Day, Memorial Day, or the Fourth of July. The fact that the veterans had many sad memories of their war experiences needed to be avoided. In addition, National Nursing Home Week was never celebrated, perhaps because to acknowledge the fact that the unit was a nursing home, within a general hospital, would also be disturbing. Another event for which there was not ritual was the death of a resident. This highly upsetting event was barely mentioned in the community. In fact, in many nursing homes this obvious and important event has no ritual. Only birthdays are celebrated! This event is in great need of a therapeutic ritual.

On the other hand, some rituals that on the surface seem to make little sense are key events in nursing homes. In the above VA nursing home, a highly charged ritual is the picnic held three blocks from the home, rather than in the backyard. The overt justification for this is that beer can be served to the veterans if they are off the grounds. Yet this means that the entire staff spends six hours moving 60 patients in small groups using one wheelchair van to the picnic site and then back again. Only a few patients actually drink beer, and the staff is left exhausted and unable to interact with the residents during the picnic. In addition, the fact that it is possible to have the doctors order beer for that day for the patients has never been pursued. This ritual therefore seems to represent a special achievement that makes this nursing home special and different from the other units at the hospital. The ritual attempts to preserve the memory of the early days of the unit, when many more veterans were younger and ambulatory. Thus, giving up this ritual, which no longer meets the unit's needs, will be to acknowledge that the unit has changed, and the good old days are gone.

NATURE OF THERAPEUTIC RITUALS

Certainly there is a role for the basic rituals of our culture (such as Christmas, birthdays) in the nursing home. These rituals are essential to maintain the link of residents to the larger culture and its traditions. However, there is also a need for the development of therapeutic rituals in the nursing home. All rituals have the therapeutic properties of strengthening the bonds of individuals to their community and in giving reassurance against the anxieties and fears of life. However, therapeutic rituals are also intentionally designed to enhance the self-esteem of the residents and the nursing home. Therapeutic rituals therefore must address issues more specific to the community of the home, and give more room for the expression of feelings among the members. These therapeutic rituals must be specifically created in each setting, and often are best designed utilizing the arts. Three particular areas of human experience around which therapeutic rituals are especially needed in the nursing home are death, achievement, and isolation.

Death. Death is of course a real presence in the nursing home, both as an event, and as part of the emotional background or context. The intensity of feeling that this issue generates makes it highly appropriate for rituals. The major rituals provided in the nursing home are birthday and anniversary celebrations. These mark the passing years and celebrate life at the same time that they acknowledge that death is closer. The actual death of a resident is another opportunity for a therapeutic ritual, one that most nursing homes do not employ, leaving the rituals (e.g., funeral, religious ceremonies) in the hands of the family. How many nursing homes have monthly ceremonies acknowledging the deaths as well as the birthdays? In VA nursing homes, Memorial Day is an excellent opportunity for a ritual concerning death, yet many do not have these ceremonies.

Nevertheless, there is a need for the staff and residents in the facility to have an organized means of dealing with the feelings around a resident's death. In the Nursing Home Care Unit at the West Haven VA, this was accomplished by creating a Remembrance Group, which meets several days after a resident's death. Like all rituals, it has a proscribed format, consisting of the leader presenting the key facts about the resident's life and how he or she died, followed by reminiscences from the patients and staff, then a moment of silence. As a therapeutic ritual, it allows for a greater amount of individual expression and encourages emotional catharsis. Not surprisingly, it is often the nursing staff, who have worked so closely with the resident for years, who have the most to say and feel the greatest sadness.

Another commonly avoided opportunity to help residents with feelings about death is the celebration of Father's and Mother's days. Usually, it is the residents who are honored, as the fathers or mothers. Yet, who are the residents thinking of on these days? *Their* fathers and mothers, who are dead. The result is a celebration that does not help residents deal with the often painful feelings of loss they are experiencing. On Father's and Mother's days, nursing homes should have ceremonies that also celebrate the memories of the residents' fathers and mothers.

Achievement. Many rituals in our culture are organized around achievements of individuals or communities. Award ceremonies, trophies, sports events, etc., all celebrate achievement, and indirectly acknowledge its partner, failure. This human need for achievement and the containment of failure is a very real issue in the nursing home, and many homes struggle hard to create meaningful rituals of achievement. The challenge is to have the achievements be real and important enough, without the underlying fears of failure to overwhelm people's awareness. Typical rituals include art shows, theatrical plays, chorus performances, award ceremonies, Veteran's Day ceremonies, and National Nursing Home Week. These activities recognize actual achievements of residents and the nursing home itself. Unfortunately, often the need to create an appearance of accomplishment undermines the meaning of the event for the resident. The fact that there are few real accomplishments of residents in the nursing home often leads to a search for substitutes. The major type is the game of chance, such as bingo, where the lucky winner psychologically feels that he or she has achieved success. In one nursing home, during their community meeting a ritual lottery is held in which a name is pulled out of a hat. The winning resident receives a dollar, and is heartily applauded. This public achievement is of great interest to the members. While reassuring, its therapeutic value remains somewhat superficial, because the image of the self is not enhanced. An example of a more therapeutic ritual of achievement that can have meaning for a nursing home community is one on the Nursing Home Care Unit, where each month certificates are given out at the community meeting for achievements in the physical therapy department. Certificates are given for best attendance, longest yards walked, and longest miles bicycled, for individuals, and then collectively for each wing. A board is posted that records cumulative distances for walking and biking. A friendly competition among residents and staff of each wing has developed that not only stimulates greater involvement in physical therapy by the residents, but creates great interest during the awards ceremony.

Isolation. Another important reality of life in the nursing home is the relative isolation from family and the wider community. This isolation is of course both disturbing and reassuring, since too much contact with visitors and the community can also be experienced as an unnecessary irritant. Nevertheless, feelings about being connected to other groups are strong, and deserve therapeutic rituals in the nursing home.

The major rituals in nursing homes concerning isolation include holiday visits from local school children, usually in the form of choral groups. Rituals may also be created around intergenerational programs, or voting in local elections. In VA nursing homes the celebration of veterans days usually brings in representatives of veterans in general, thereby acknowledging the residents' links to a larger community.

A significant gap in therapeutic rituals exists around family contacts, which are often as disturbing as they are welcomed by both residents and staff. Most communities have rituals that symbolize feelings of isolation from family members such as Parent's Days at summer camps and colleges, which handle the students' homesickness and the parents' curiosity. This ritual also serves to protect the integrity of the community—channeling what would otherwise be irritating and unpredictable intrusions from parents. In the nursing home, a number of ritual events could be created to express and organize the feelings associated with family contacts, such as Family Night, Family Recognition Day, or·Family Bingo. These events would serve to protect the nursing home from the otherwise relentless, unpredictable intrusion of family members. The ritual would offer time for individuals to express their gratitude for being a part of a family. Of course, this will highlight the fact that some residents do not have any living family. Thus a therapeutic family ritual needs to include a structure for celebrating the families of the past as well as the present.

The issues of death, achievement, and isolation are three key foci around which therapeutic rituals can be constructed. The challenge is to create a ritual that is safe enough and yet allows for the expression of the disturbing, upsetting emotions that it represents. The ritual event needs to be both emotionally close to the actual issues so that it is felt to be meaningful and authentic, and yet distant enough not to overwhelm the participants with distressing emotion. This combination of transparency and distance is present in aesthetic distance, in the forms of expression of the arts. Aesthetic distance transforms the inner world of intense feeling into a perception of beauty. Aesthetic distance allows a sculpture of a naked woman to be beautiful and not sexually arousing. This transformation is the result of the process of symbolization, in which feeling is both preserved and altered (Langer, 1953). It is this intimate link between the arts and internal experience that gives the arts their special relationship to healing (Scheff, 1979). For this reason, therapeutic rituals are often best designed using the methods of the creative arts therapies. The following example describes one attempt to create such a ritual that deals with the issue of isolation.

CASE EXAMPLE

I will now describe how a therapeutic ritual was developed to address a specific situation in a nursing home.

Background

The New Haven Convalescent Center (NHCC) is an 89-bed general nursing home whose backyard joins the field behind the Barnard Elementary school. The NHCC consists mostly of white middle-class Protestants and Catholics, while the school is attended by urban, lower class black children. For two years an intergenerational program was developing between these two facilities, in an attempt to link the nursing home with the community and to link the children with the elderly. Many of the black nursing aide staff lived in the area, and their children attended Barnard. This intergenerational program is described in chapters 10 and 11 of this book.

The intergenerational program had been a great success, in that the children had become comfortable with the elderly residents, and were even showing up after school to visit with them. The elderly patients had gone over to the school several times to perform with their choral group, and to participate in several joint activities. Nevertheless, the program generated its own strains; the teachers and principal had to deal with more complex programming in order to bring the children over to the nursing home; precious NHCC staff time was taken up in scheduling programs and negotiating with the school; the children were often loud when they came, distracting nursing staff, and bothering some residents. The positive and negative aspects of linking with the wider community were apparent, and created tension. One problem was that the administrator (Sandel) was perceived as spearheading and representing the values of the intergenerational program, so that the negative attitudes initially did not have an official spokesperson. Finally, these attitudes did emerge when the patients angrily requested to have their own bingo, where children would not be allowed. The administrator agreed to this. The need for a containing ritual or ceremonial event to mark the importance of the intergenerational program, and more generally the new relationship between the school and the nursing home, was now more evident.

The Primary Image: The Gate

When the nursing home had been built, a ten-foot high chain link fence had been erected between the home and the school. As a result, the children and the elderly residents needed to be brought around the block to visit for intergenerational programs. This was especially tiresome for the nursing home staff who had to push the patients in their wheelchairs. The idea finally occurred to the staff to build a gate in the fence, so that the patients and children had more direct access to each other. The gate could be locked after school hours to maintain security. The plans for this gate were being developed as the school year was coming to a close. The real and symbolic meaning of this Intergenerational Gate, that of bringing the old and young together, seemed to be a perfect vehicle for a ritual ceremony that would also mark the end of the year's programming. Thus the primary image for the ritual became the opening of a way between the generations, not an elimination of boundaries, but the creation of a controllable gate in what had been an impenetrable wall.

The Preparation

The design team consisted of the author as the director, and members of the NHCC and Barnard school. The elements of the ceremony were based on three concepts: (1) that everyone participate in some manner, (2) that it be held outdoors in the field, and (3) that the format be essentially an artistic one, with song, drama, music, and costumes. The participants were divided into four major groups: the children, the elderly, guests (family, friends, and community), and the artists who orchestrated the event. Each group would be represented on stage by a spokesperson—the principal, the administrator, the Mayor of New Haven, and the director, respectively. The ceremony would take place at noon, and be followed by a picnic lunch. With 250 children, 100 patients, 50 artists, 50 staff and teachers, and 100 guests, the event would indeed be a large one.

The author had been impressed with the work of the Bread and Puppet Theatre, under the direction of Peter Schumann, who developed methods of communal ritual that include large puppets carried by 2-5 people, representing archetypal figures and forces relevant to particular issues and communities (e.g., nuclear war, oppression). A ceremony was designed using this model, with two 15 foot high puppets, one representing youth, and the other old age. The Child and the Elder were two Great Spirits, who would be called up by the participants and then enact a therapeutic story concerning the old and young. The actual dedication of the Intergenerational Gate would be the culminating event of the ceremony. The author called upon the network of artists and creative arts therapists in New Haven to be puppet builders, puppeteers, banner carriers, story tellers, musicians, and costumed members of the puppet parade. Large 15-foot square banners with the profiles of a child and an older person were created, to be draped from each building. The nursing home prepared to feed 500 people, and the city of New Haven prepared the field and provided police coverage. Local businesses were asked to donate sound equipment, chairs, and parking space. The school and nursing home became acutely aware of their newly acquired public status.

The structure of the ceremony was based on dividing up the groups into manageable units, so that the children could be controlled and the contribution of each subgroup could be better articulated. Special education teachers and therapists with an interest in the arts volunteered to work with each of the ten classes of students. These "team leaders" visited their assigned class twice before the event to orient them to the ceremony, teach them the communal song, and develop their own chant and decorate their own flags. In the actual ceremony, each subgroup (school class, guests, and the elderly patients) was led by a Team Leader, a banner carrier, and a teacher. Only the Team Leaders and banner carriers rehearsed the choreography and content of the ceremony with the Director, so that the day of the ceremony was the first time that the children, elderly, and guests experienced the ritual. They were instructed to follow the cues of their Team Leader, who was in turn cued by the Director from the stage in the middle of the field. Using this system, a rather complicated ritual was developed without taking inordinate time from school or nursing home activities.

The Ceremony

Preparations went smoothly. The field was laid out with a raised platform at one end, the children's classes (called the Young) in separate groups; to the left of the stage, the group of guests (called Adults) in the center, and the elderly patients (called the Old) on a hill in front of the nursing home, to the right of the platform. They were on the other side of the chain link fence from the children. The puppets, musical bands and costumed people were out of sight several hundred yards away. The ceremony consists of five sections: Greeting, Calling Up the Spirits, Opening the Gate, a Story, and the Exit.

OPEN THE GATE RITUAL CEREMONY

Greeting

	(Trumpet blast. Entrance of mayor, principal, administrator and special guests, surrounded by ten banner carriers.)
Singer:	(Begins song about happiness.)
Old:	(In unison, slowly wave one hand to the Young.)
Young:	(In unison, they wave back to the Old with flags in their hands. Guests walk onto stage, banner carriers move to their assigned classes. Quiet.)
Master of Ceremonies:	The hour of noon is upon us. The generations have gathered. Our banners are unfurled. We are ready.
	(Clock strikes noon).
Old:	Hello children! (In unison, waving their hands).
Young:	Hello old ones, wise ones!
Adults:	(To the Old) Hello to our parents!
	(To the Young) Hello to our children!
Young:	(To Adults) Hello to our parents!
Old:	(To Adults) Hello to our children!
Young:	(To Adults) Is this our day?

Adults:	Yes, this is your day.
Old:	(To Adults) Is this our day?
Adults:	Yes, this is your day.
	You have our Blessing, you have our Blessing!
MC:	So let the ceremony begin!
	This fence has stood between these two places for many years.
	This—a house for the old. This—a house for the young.
	Their backs to each other.
	Today, a Gate will open in this fence,
	allowing the old and young to touch each other.
	We have come to dedicate this gate.
	(To Old) What do you say?
Old:	Open the Gate!
MC:	(To Young) What do you say?
Young:	(Each class chants one at a time, each with its own variation)
	Open the Gate!
MC:	And what do you say?
Adults:	Open the Gate!
MC:	What do we all say?
Singer:	(Leads everyone in the ritual song, which is accompanied by a set of arm gestures that children and patients have already learned.)
	Open the gate. Open it wide.
	Reach across the ages with your hand.
	Here are the old. Here are the young.
	Bring them all together in your heart. (Repeat)

Calling Up the Spirits

MC:	Let us now call up the Great Spirits, to help us open the way between the generations. Let us wave our flags and sing out, ''Ohhhh!''
All:	Ohhhh!
Old:	(As the Elder Puppet and accompanying band arrive over the crest of a hill and enter the field:)
	Here comes the Elder, the one who holds the Past!
	(Young wave their flags, Adults applaud, and the Puppet waves back.)

Young: (As the Child Puppet enters from the other side of the field:)
              Here comes the Child, the one who holds the Future!
              (Old wave, Adults applaud, and the Puppet waves.)

MC: Here they come! The Elder will lead us in the Intergenerational Parade. (Everyone moves around the field led by the Puppets, as the Singer sings another song. At the end, everyone returns and the puppets move to either side of the Gate.)

Opening the Gate

              (Trumpet blast)
MC: Hear ye. Hear ye.
              Let all who are now present behold.
              The bond created between young and old.
              Men and women of great station
              Have come to this gate dedication.
              First the Lord Mayor of New Haven
              Who will make a proclamation!

Mayor: *Whereas*: Your exciting and truly meaningful Intergenerational Program brings together young and old in an atmosphere of love and affection and sharing; and
              Whereas: We have gathered here today to dedicate this Intergenerational Gate which symbolizes the wonderful relationship between young and old;
              Therefore, I, Mayor of the City of New Haven, do hereby proclaim today as *Intergenerational Gate Dedication Day*!

MC: And now, the Grand Administrator of the New Haven Convalescent Center, and the High Principal of Barnard Elementary
              each to the other, a living plant they will trade,
              to show their hope for the future
              and friendship that will never fade.
              (They trade plants).

MC: The Ambassadors from New Haven Convalescent

Center and Barnard Elementary, Julia and Carmel,
will now read us their poems
written from the heart,
each filled with spirit.
(Julia, a resident of the nursing home, and Carmel, a fourth grader, had each prepared an original poem for the ceremony.)

Julia: Let us open the gates to Barnard School,
And welcome the young into our hearts and thoughts.
We communicate, we share, we feel, and we touch.
The hearts of the old begin to throb,
The eyes of the young gleam with joy,
The day ends with dreams of the past and hopes of the future.

Carmel: The young and the old are like two flowers:
To me, the young are a small flower bud.
As they grow older, they grow bigger and sweeter.
To me, the old are a big wide open flower,
As big and wide as a flower can be.
But as flowers wither, people die,
And we will always remember them in our hearts,
For when each were here,
They made the world more beautiful.

MC: And now are we ready?

All: READY!

MC: Let us turn toward the Gate, where the Great Spirits are.

Old: Open the Gate!

Young: Open the Gate!

Adults: What is there to fear?

Old: Let us touch you.

Young: Let us hug you.

Adult: There is nothing to fear.

(Puppets hug each other, bands play to a crescendo, and a huge helium balloon is released as the Gate is swung open. Attached to the balloon is a ribbon connected to each building.)

MC:	The Gate is open!
Old:	The Gate is open!
Young:	The Gate is open!
Adult:	The Gate is open!
MC:	Let the Banners unfurl. (Banners with profiles of old and young are released from the roof of each building. Singer sings.)

The Story

MC:	Wait! The Great Spirits are going to tell us a story, which will surely reveal a great truth, since they are so wise. We will need the great wizard of New Haven to translate their message.
Wizard:	(Narrates this story as the puppets, and a man on stilts representing Mr. Responsible, enact the story in front of the crowd.)

Once upon a time in a place far away, there lived a man named Mr. Responsible. Mr. Responsible had a parent who was very very old. Mr. Responsible was very concerned about this parent. He didn't know what to do. So he put his parent in a very special room, which was set up for very old people. Mr. Responsible also had a child, who was very very young. He was very concerned about his child also, and he didn't know what to do. So he designed a very special room on the other side of the house for this child, which was set up for the very young. For a while Mr. Responsible thought everything was all right, since both his parent and his child had their own very special rooms, set up for the old and the young.

Every day Mr. Responsible visited his parent's room. And he became very very concerned. He thought his parent didn't look so well, so he took a pulse. Then he remembered his child, and he rushed over to the child's room, and read him a story. When this child didn't seem to listen, he became very very concerned.

On other days, Mr. Responsible worried that

his parent was running a fever. So he insisted on taking a temperature, which his parent definitely did not like. And then he ran to the other room, because he had forgotten to give his child the weekly allowance, which his child definitely wanted.

Back and forth, Mr. Responsible went, taking care of his parent and his child. Poor Mr. Responsible! He didn't seem to satisfy anybody, and he was wearing himself out. He would run up to his parent's room, and quickly shout, "Looking good today!" while his parent politely nodded. "But I have to go take care of Johnny, see you soon." And he would be off to his child's room, to scold him for misbehaving. He did that so often.

Mr. Responsible became more and more concerned, and more and more responsible, and more and more tired out. "But I can't stop," he cried, "what would each do without me?" Finally the day came when Mr. Responsible could not get up out of bed. He was simply too exhausted to rise. He was even too exhausted to be concerned about his parent and his child.

His parent and his child waited for him to come. When he didn't, they tiptoed out of their special rooms, set up for the very old and the very young. They met each other in the living room. "Where have you been?" the grandparent asked the child. "In my special room," said the child, "And where have *you* been?" "In my special room," said the grandparent. All afternoon the grandparent and child played together; they had a great time. They did not need a special room.

Finally, they went together to Mr. Responsible's bedroom. Mr. Responsible was shocked to see them out of their very special rooms, which had been designed for them. "Mr. Responsible," they said, "We thank you for taking care of us, for your concern for us. But you cannot do it alone. Join us and each of us can learn to care for one another. In that way the burden will be shared."

	Mr. Responsible took their hands, and all three faced the concerns of life together. The next day Mr. Responsible built another special room, one designed for all three generations; the very very young, the very very old, and the very very responsible.
All:	(Applause, as Puppets bow and begin to leave.)

Departure

MC:	The Great Spirits are leaving us now. Wave good-bye to them.
Old:	Goodbye Great Ones.
Young:	Goodbye Great Ones.
Adults:	Goodbye Great Ones.
	(Bands play as the puppets exit, Singer sings a farewell song.)
MC:	(Cues Old, Young, and Adults who wave slowly to the Puppets, then to each other, as Singer finishes her song.)
MC:	Our ceremony is ended. See you next year.

Follow-Up

The intergenerational gate ceremony has become a yearly ritual for the New Haven Convalescent Center and the Barnard Elementary school. Each year in the late spring the ritual is performed. Both institutions include it in their calendar of expected events. It clearly serves to anchor and concretize a developing relationship that has affected each one deeply. The format remains essentially the same, though the content continues to transform each year to more accurately represent the most salient issues. The gate ceremony has even expanded now to include other nursing homes and other schools, the "gate" now representing the connections that can be created among a wider range of community institutions. At the heart of it remain the puppets, the chants, the "open the gate" song, and the therapeutic stories enacted in the ritual. The essence of this ritual lies in its representation of the ambivalent feelings associated with opening oneself to another. Its therapeutic power as a community ritual is based on both the joy and the fear of bringing the old and young together. Due to this ambivalence, the ritual event has the opportunity to be the vehicle for institutional change and transformation. Both NHCC and Barnard were relatively isolated institutions, both with marginal self-esteem. Without question, the creation and enactment of the gate ritual has increased their self-esteem.

Impact on the School

The ceremony seemed to crystallize for the children a set of feelings and ideas that the entire intergenerational program had engendered. The link with another group of people seemed to be reassuring and protective. The children adopted many of the elements of the ritual: the song, characters from the story and puppets, and flags. For months after the ceremony, the children were heard singing the "open the gate" song while coming to school. The after-school visits by the children increased. An after-school intergenerational bowling was established to accommodate this increased interest.

Establishing this level of trust and intimacy with the children has made its demands on the nursing home. As the years have progressed, the children have begun to use the nursing home as a means of seeking help. Several children have told nursing staff about problems at home, including alcoholism, child abuse, and hunger. Often staff and residents have become quite involved. Deciding when it is appropriate to intervene has become a challenge to the administration of the nursing home. How much easier it would be if there was no connection between these facilities! These complexities are the price of a relationship; attention and care must be given continuously in order for it to be sustained. Fortunately the benefits of this relationship between NHCC and Barnard are clear: the children have incorporated the message of the gate ceremony and the intergenerational programming, and the ritual is eagerly awaited each year.

Impact on the Nursing Home

The nursing home has also been transformed by the program and the institution of the ritual ceremony. The presence of Barnard children in the facility is now taken for granted, though they are both a joy and a bother, as are all children.

The facility had previously identified itself as a tightknit entity, "like a family." There is evidence that the ritual has changed that identity. Shortly after the ritual, the aides and other staff groups developed links with workers in other facilities. Interestingly, a key leader in this effort was the activities worker most involved with the gate ceremony, and the most committed to the administrator's vision of linking with the community. By the end of the summer following the gate ceremony, the atmosphere in the nursing home had radically changed. Not only was the facility now linked to the Barnard school and the immediate community, but its own workers had altered the exclusive "family" link with the facility and had connected with their own wider community. The process begun in the intergenerational programming, and concretized in the gate ceremony, had led to a significant transformation of the nursing home environment. It was now more connected to the world, but it had given up some of its protective insularity and closeknit feeling. This change continues to be ambivalently experienced by both patients and staff.

Conclusion

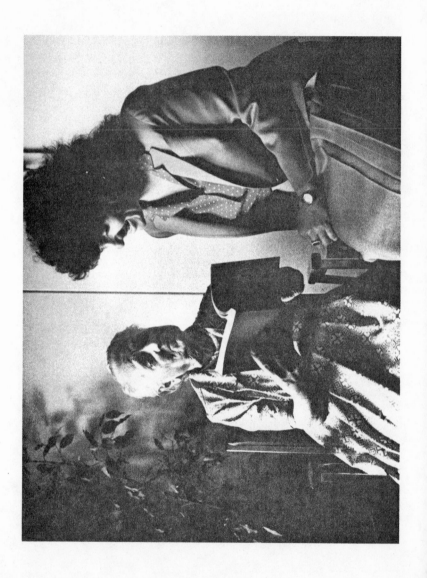

The Gate

Before one goes through the gate
one may not be aware there is a gate
One may think there is a gate to go through
and look a long time for it
without finding it
One may find it and
it may not open
If it opens one may be through it
As one goes through it
one sees that the gate one went through
was the self that went through it
no one went through a gate
there was not a gate to go through
no one ever found a gate
no one ever realized there was never a gate

R. D. Laing, *Knots* (1970)

What is the gate? What does it symbolize? In this book we have talked about many gates. The gate of the nurses' station. The gates of heaven. The gate between the nursing home and the school. The gates between people, and the gates within the self.

As a metaphor, the gate marks the boundary between two states of being. It represents a transformation of the self in which the self changes, and yet stays the same. One is not a different person, but one is different.

A living organism is an open system with a boundary and an internal organization which carries on transactions with the environment (von Bertalanffy, 1968). A dead organism, in contrast, is a closed system. Our work with older people and the institutions in which they live focuses on sustaining these transactions across boundaries in order to maintain living rather than dying systems, and to counteract the unnecessary fall towards stasis and paralysis. Our experiences with nursing home residents have taught us that an environment that supports creative activity, expressive interaction, physical vitality and spontaneity can be a growth-promoting and enlivening place to be. The healing community transforms passive receiving into mutual giving, inactivity into purposeful motion, and waiting into creating. We believe that the nursing home can be transformed into a healing community when the values of creativity, playfulness, and honesty in the acknowledgement of human emotions are supported by the administration and implemented in programs by a skilled and caring staff. Such efforts challenge the phenomenon of the custodial nursing home, and offer creative alternatives to elders who seek communal residential care.

Our efforts have led us to open the gates between institutions of the young and the old through the intergenerational programs, to open the gates between people through our group therapy programs, and to open the gates between past and present aspects of the self through our work with life review, reminiscence and insight. Maintaining a flow of information and communication back and forth, in and out, is essential to living.

And what better way to do this than through the arts! For the arts themselves refer to multiple levels of reality; they are concrete and present, yet they are also abstract and transcendent. Because the arts are symbolic, they are excellent vehicles for travelling through intangible gates. By giving access to the imagination and the unconscious, the arts allow us to travel through time, to the past or the future, to speak with others who cannot speak, to understand those who do not share our language.

Movement and drama in particular offer powerful means for these transformations of self. Physical movement becomes a metaphor for *inner* movement, and theatrical enactment becomes a symbol for the dramatic story of our lives. These performing arts revitalize time because they rely on the dynamics of pulse, rhythm, and development. They are thus antidotes to timelessness, immobility, and death—the spawning ground for hoplessness and despair.

Not that death can be or should be avoided. Each of us will pass through the final Gate. But to pass through that gate well, and to approach that final transformation of spirit, it is better to have been open to the world, to others, and to oneself. That is what we believe. That is what we have found.

References

Abraham, K. (1949). The applicability of psychoanalytic treatment for patients at an advanced age. *Selected papers on psychoanalysis*. London: Hogarth Press.

Almond, R. (1974). *The healing community*. New York: Jason Aronson.

American Association of Homes for the Aging. (1985). *Guide to caring for the mentally impaired elderly*. Washington: Author.

Bartenieff, I. (1972). Dance therapy: A new profession or a rediscovery of an ancient role of the dance? *Dance Scope*, *7*, 6-18.

Benaim, S. (1957). Group psychotherapy within a geriatric unit: An experiment. *International Journal of Social Psychiatry*, *3*, 123-128.

Berezin, M. (1969). Sex and old age: A review of the literature. *Journal of Geriatric Psychiatry*, *2*, 131-149.

Berger, E. (1985). The institutionalization of patients with Alzheimer's disease. *Nursing Homes*, *34*, 22-29.

Berger, L., & Berger, M. (1973). A holistic group approach to psychogeriatric outpatients. *International Journal of Group Psychotherapy*, *23*, 432-444.

Berland, D., & Poggi, R. (1979). Expressive group psychotherapy with the aging. *International Journal of Group Psychotherapy*, *29*, 87-109.

von Bertalanffy, L. (1968). *General system theory*. New York: Braziller.

Boling, T.E. (1984). A new image of long-term care: Challenge to management. *Long Term Care Administration*, *12*, 15-17.

Bortz, W. (1981). Effect of exercise on aging—effect of aging on exercise. *American Geriatrics Society*, *28*, 49-51.

Bruner, J. (1964). The course of cognitive growth. *American Psychologist*, *19*, 1-15.

Burger, I. (1981). *Creative drama for senior adults*. Wilton, CT: Morehouse Barlow Co.

Butler, R. (1963). The life review: An interpretation of reminiscence in the aged. *Psychiatry*, *26*, 65-75.

Butler, R. (1974). Successful aging and the role of the life review. *Journal of the American Geriatrics Society*, *22*, 529-535.

Butler, R. (1975). *Why survive? Being old in America*. New York: Harper & Row.

Butler, R. (1981). The teaching nursing home. *Journal of the American Medical Association*, *245*, 1435-1437.

Butler, R., & Lewis, M. (1973). *Aging and mental health*. St. Louis: C.V. Mosby.

Caplow-Lindner, E., Harpaz, L., & Samberg, S. (1979). *Therapeutic dance movement: Expressive activities for older adults*. New York: Human Sciences Press.

Chace, M. (1975). *Marian Chace: Her papers*, (H. Chaiklin, Ed.). Columbia, MD: American Dance Therapy Association.

Chaiklin, S., & Schmais, C. (1975). Dance therapy. In S. Arieti (Ed.), *American handbook of psychiatry* (Chapter 37). New York: Basic Books.

Chaiklin, S., & Schmais, C. (1979). Chace approach to dance therapy. In P. Bernstein (Ed.), *Eight theoretical approaches in dance-movement therapy*, (pp. 15-30). Davenport, Iowa: Kendall Hunt.

Cole, D. (1975). *The theatrical event*. Middletown, CT: Wesleyan University Press.

Cook, J. (1981). Rate your APE (activity producing environment). *American Health Care Association Journal*, *7*, 18-20.

Crossin, C. (1976). Art therapy with geriatric patients: Problems of spontaneity. *American Journal of Art Therapy*, *15*, 35-58.

Cummings, J., & Cummings, E. (1962). *Ego and milieu: Theory and practice of environmental therapy*. New York: Atherton.

deVries, H. (1974). Education for physical fitness in the later years. In S. Grabowski & W. Mason (Eds.), *Learning for aging*, Washington, DC: Adult Education Association.

Dewdney, I. (1973). An art therapy program for geriatric patients. *American Journal of Art Therapy, 12*, 249-254.

Edelson, M. (1970). *Sociotherapy and psychotherapy*. Chicago: University of Chicago Press.

Erickson, E. (1968). *Identity: youth and crisis*. New York: Norton.

Fallot, R.D. (1976). *The life story through reminiscence in later adulthood*. Unpublished doctoral dissertation, Yale University Department of Psychology.

Feil, N. (1981). *Validation-fantasy therapy*. Cleveland: Feil Productions.

Fersh, I. (1980). Dance/movement therapy: A holistic approach to working with the elderly. *American Journal of Dance Therapy, 3*, 33-43.

Fogelberg, T. (1985). A resident's view on living the nursing home life. *American Health Care Association Journal, 11*, 52-53.

Fowke, E. (1969). *Sally go round the sun, 300 children's songs, rhymes, and games*. Garden City, NY: Doubleday.

Fowke, E., & Seeger, R.C. (1948). *American folk songs for children*. Garden City, NY: Doubleday.

Freud, S. (1962). On psychotherapy. In J. Strachey (Ed.), *The standard edition of the complete psychological works of Sigmund Freud* (Vol. 7, pp. 257-270). London: Hogarth Press. (Original work published 1905.)

Freud, S. (1962). Humour. In J. Strachey (Ed.), *The standard edition of the complete psychological works of Sigmund Freud* (Vol. 21, pp. 160-167). London: Hogarth Press. (Original work published in 1927.)

Garnet, E.D. (1972). Geriatric calisthenics: A group therapy approach. *Writings on body movement and communication. Monograph No. 2*. Columbia, MD: American Dance Therapy Association.

Goldfarb, A. (1953). Recommendations for psychiatric care in a home for the aged. *Journal of Gerontology, 8*, 343-347.

Gray, P. (1974). *Dramatics for the elderly*. New York: Teachers College, Columbia University Press.

Gulton, L. (1975). *Don't give up on an aging patient*. New York: Crown Publishing.

Guntrip, H. (1961). *Personality structure and human interaction*. New York: International Universities Press.

Hellebrandt, F.A. (1978). Comment: The senile dement in our midst. *The Gerontologist, 18*, 67-70.

Herman, G., & Renzurri, J. (1978). *Creative movement for older people*. Hartford, CT: Institute for Movement Exploration.

Irwin, E. Baker, N., & Bloom, L. (1976). Fantasy, play, and language: Expressive therapy with communication handicapped children. *Journal of Childhood Communication Disorders, 1*, 99-115.

Irwin, K. (1972). Dance as a prevention of, therapy for, and recreation from the crisis of old age. *Writings on body movement and communication. Monograph No. 2*. Columbia, MD: American Dance Therapy Association.

Jennings, S. (1973). *Remedial drama*. London: Pitman.

Johnson, D. (1981a). Drama therapy and the schizophrenic condition. In G. Schattner & R. Courtney (Eds.), *Drama in therapy*, (Vol. 2, pp. 47-66). New York: Drama Book Specialists.

Johnson, D. (1981b). Some diagnostic implications of drama therapy. In G. Schattner & R. Courtney (Eds.), *Drama in therapy*, (Vol. 2, pp. 13-35). New York: Drama Book Specialists.

Johnson, D. (1982a). Developmental approaches in drama therapy. *International Journal of Arts in Psychotherapy, 9*, 172-181.

Johnson, D. (1982b). Principles and techniques of drama therapy. *International Journal of Arts in Psychotherapy, 9*, 83-90.

Johnson, D. (1984). Representation of the internal world in catatonic schizophrenia. *Psychiatry, 47*, 299-314.

Johnson, D. (1985). Envisioning the links among the creative arts therapies. *International Journal of Arts in Psychotherapy, 12*, 233-238.

Johnson, D., Sandel, S., & Eicher, V. (1983). Structural aspects of group leadership styles. *American Journal of Dance Therapy, 6*, 17-30.

Jones, M. (1953). *The therapeutic community.* New York: Basic Books.

Keelor, R. (1976). *The role of physical fitness in reducing health problems and long-term care of the elderly.* Testimony to the joint hearing held by Subcommittees on Health and Long-Term Care, Federal, State and Community Relations, and the Select Committee on Aging. Washington, DC: United States Congress.

Kelleher, M. (1978). *Social interaction and affective expression in group movement therapy with the elderly.* Unpublished masters thesis, Wesleyan University, Middletown, CT.

Kernberg, O. (1976). *Object relations theory and clinical psychoanalysis.* New York: Aronson.

Klein, M. (1975). *Writings of Melanie Klein. Vols. 1-3.* London: Hogarth.

Klein, T. (1979). Psycho-opera. Presentation at the annual meeting of the American Society of Group Psychotherapy and Psychodrama, New York.

Kraus, H. (1956). *Principles and practice of therapeutic exercise.* Springfield, Ill.: Charles Thomas.

Kübler-Ross, E. (1969). *On death and dying.* New York: Macmillan.

Laing, R.D. (1970). *Knots.* New York: Random House.

Langer, S. (1953). *Feeling and form.* New York: Scribner's.

Levine, J. (1977). Humor as a form of therapy. In A. Chapman & H. Foot (Eds.), *It's a Funny Thing, Humor* (pp. 219-243). London: Pergamon Press.

Lewis, C.N. (1971). Reminiscence and self-concept in old age. *Journal of Gerontology, 26*, 240-243.

Linden, M.E. (1953). Group psychotherapy with institutionalized senile women: Studies in gerontologic human relations. *International Journal of Group Psychotherapy, 3*, 150-170.

Linden, M. (1954). The significance of dual leadership in gerontologic group psychotherapy: Studies in gerontologic human relations. *International Journal of Group Psychotherapy, 4*, 262-273.

Linden, M.E. (1955). Transference in gerontologic group psychotherapy: Studies in gerontologic human relations. *International Journal of Group Psychotherapy, 5*, 61-79.

Linden, M. (1956). Geriatrics. In S. Slavson (Ed.), *Fields of group psychotherapy*, (pp. 129-152). New York: International Universities Press.

McMahon, A.W., & Rhudick, P.J. (1967). Reminiscing in the aged: An adaptational response. In S. Levin & R. Kahana (Eds.), *Psychodynamic studies on aging*, (pp. 64-78). New York: International Universities Press.

McNiff, S. (1981). *The arts and psychotherapy.* Springfield: Charles Thomas.

Meerloo, J. (1955). Transference and resistance in geriatric psychotherapy. *Psychoanalytic Review, 42*, 72-82.

Michaels, C. (1981). Geriadrama. In G. Schattner & R. Courtney (Eds.), *Drama in therapy*, (Vol. 2, pp. 175-196). New York: Drama Book Specialists.

Mosey, A. (1973). *Activities therapy.* New York: Raven Press.

Needler, W., & Baer, M. (1982). Movement, music and remotivation with the regressed elderly. *Journal of Gerontological Nursing, 8*, 497-503.

Nelson, E. (1977). *Musical games for children.* New York: Sterling.

Oberleder, M. (1966). Psychotherapy with the aging: An art of the possible? *Psychotherapy: Theory, Research, & Practice, 3*, 139-142.

Oliphant, R. (1985). The American nursing home: A novelist's view. *Nursing Homes, 34*, 20.

Piaget, J. (1951). *Play, dreams, and imitation in childhood.* New York: Norton.

Rechtschaffen, A. (1959). Psychotherapy with geriatric patients: A review of the literature. *Gerontology*, *14*, 73-84.

Riesman, D. (1950). *The lonely crowd*. New Haven: Yale University Press.

Robbins, A. (1980). *Expressive therapy: A creative arts approach to depth-oriented treatment*. New York: Human Sciences Press.

Rowen, B. (1963). *Learning through movement*. New York: Teachers College, Columbia University Press.

Samuels, A. (1973). Dance therapy for geriatric patients. *Proceedings of the Eighth Annual Conference of the American Dance Therapy Association*, *8*, 27-30.

Sandel, S. (1980). Dance therapy in the psychiatric hospital. *Journal of the Association of Private Psychiatric Hospitals*, *11*, 20-26.

Sandel, S., & Johnson D. (1983). Structure and process of the nascent group: Dance therapy with chronic patients. *International Journal of Arts in Psychotherapy*, *10*, 131-140.

Schattner, G., & Courtney, R. (1981). *Drama in therapy, Vols. I and II*. New York: Drama Book Specialists.

Scheff, T. (1979). *Catharsis in healing, ritual, and drama*. Berkeley: University of California Press.

Schimek, J. (1975). A critical re-examination of Freud's concept of unconscious mental representation. *International Review of Psychoanalysis*, *2*, 171-187.

Schwartz, E., & Goodman, J. (1952). Group therapy of obesity in elderly diabetics. *Geriatrics*, *7*, 280-283.

Searles, H. (1977). The development of mature hope in the patient-therapist relationship. In K. Frank (Ed.), *The human dimension in psychoanalytic practice*, (pp. 9-27). New York: Grune & Stratton.

Shaw, A. (1980). *Drama, theatre, and the handicapped*. Washington, DC: American Theatre Association.

Shere, E.S. (1964). Group therapy with the very old. In R. Kastenbaum (Ed.), *New thoughts on old age*, (pp. 146-160). New York: Springer.

Silver, A. (1950). Group psychotherapy with senile psychotic patients. *Geriatrics*, *5*, 147-150.

Slater, P. (1970). *The pursuit of loneliness*. Boston: Beacon Press.

Spalding, J., & Frank, B. (1985). Quality care from the resident's point of view. *American Health Care Association Journal*, *2*, 3-7.

Sterns, E. (1947, June). Buried alive. *Women's Home Companion*.

Thurman, A., & Piggins, C. (1982). *Drama activities for elders: A handbook for leaders*. New York: The Haworth Press.

Verwoerdt, A. (1976). *Clinical geropsychiatry*. Baltimore: Williams & Wilkins.

Weisberg, N., & Wilder, R. (1985). *Creative arts with older adults*. New York: Human Sciences Press.

Weiss, J. (1984). *Expressive therapy with elders and the disabled*. New York: The Haworth Press.

Werner, H. (1948). *Comparative psychology of mental development*. New York: International Universities Press.

Werner, H., & Kaplan, S. (1964). *Symbol formation*. New York: Wiley.

Winnicott, D. (1953). Transitional objects and transitional phenomena. *International Journal of Psycho-analysis*, *34*, 89-97.

Winnicott, D. (1971). *Playing and reality*. New York: Basic Books.

Wolff, K. (1963). *Geriatric psychiatry*. Springfield, IL: Charles Thomas.

Yalom, I. (1975). *Theory and practice of group psychotherapy*. New York: Basic Books.

Zieger, B. (1976). Life review in art therapy with the aged. *American Journal of Art Therapy*, *15*, 34-45.

Ziemba, J. (1985). *Drama and plays for the older thespian*. Agawam, MA: Educational Parameters.

Index